ANTI-AGING SECRETS

The Complete Self-Rejuvenation Manual for Conscious Men and Women

by

Mahayana Isabelle Dugast
Ph.D.

Strategic Book Group

Strategic Book Group
P.O. Box 333
Durham CT 06422
www.StrategicBookClub.com

ISBN:978-1-60976-899-7

Warning-Disclaimer

The material in this book should not replace advice or treatment by your healthcare provider. This book presents information based on ancient knowledge and cosmetic procedures. All matters linked to your health require medical supervision from the health practitioner of your choice. People have different levels of awareness and the adoption and application of the material offered in this book must be your own responsibility. Neither the publisher nor the author accept any legal responsibility for any personal injury or other damage or loss arising from the use or misuse of the information and advice offered in this book.

This book is dedicated to

YOU, the Gatekeeper of your life and the Guardian of your body, mind, and soul,
which is a magnificent work of art and one of the most intricate reflections of the Divine.
This book is a gift to you,
and is intended as a refinement tool to promote peaceful living in health, beauty and harmony.
May it contribute to your greater realization of who you truly are,
and assist you in increasing your natural state of abundance.

Real success unfolds from within…

TABLE OF CONTENTS

Chapter Three

Chapter Four

Chapter Five

APPENDIX

ACKNOWLEDGMENTS

A myriad of faces come to mind now and I would like to express my gratitude to all those from whom I have learned—an eclectic mix of men and women working within their chosen field: medical doctors, complementary practitioners, spiritual teachers (from both the East and West), shamans, business men and women, and friends and family in physical and spiritual form.

With all my heart, I want to express my humble gratitude to the following friends, who generously found time to help me with this project in spite of their incredibly busy lives. I would like to thank:

Mary McCarthy, who generously offered her professional advice and positive belief in this project while still in its infancy; Eoin McCuirc, a good friend and a multitalented natural healer; and Elizabeth Collins, a close and faithful friend for many years. I am also deeply grateful to Dorothy O'Regan, who has been a supportive and motivating force in this project, and Lavinia Hartigan, for her time and valued contribution. I also thank Jane Skovgaard for her artistic talent in illustrating some of the exercises described in this book. Special thanks to Maria Mackessy for her inspirational teachings, Soizic Nogues for her support, James McKeon for his shared experience at writing and publishing, and Noel Ahern for his insight and contributions.

I wish to express my gratitude to Dr. T. Chang and The Great Tao Foundation for their permission in letting me use "The Tummy Rubbing Exercise," extracted from *The Complete System of Self-Healing: Internal Exercises*, a book full of gems that should absolutely be read by anyone seriously wishing to make the most of their body-temple!

I thank Rosemary Moone for teaching me her valuable insights on the Alexander Technique, which she has been practicing for many years. She has kindly allowed me to use her illustration, "The constructive rest position," for which I am most grateful.

Last but definitely not least, thanks go to my three amazing sons: Azaro, Sudesh, and Imralis, without whom none of this would have happened. Thank you for putting up with me at times when I got totally googly-eyed due to long hours spent glued to my computer; you had to cook your own meals … and mine! The four of us weave our dreams into reality through the powerful love, strength, and respect that we share, and the fun we have! Always present to remind each other that we believe in one another, especially when we lose sight of it. I am a lucky mum!

INTRODUCTION

Whether you would like to enhance and keep your youthful appearance, or are concerned with good health and an increase of your potential: this book is for you!

The truth is that health and beauty are closely linked, as they reflect one another. So we are going to explore each and every possible way to age gracefully, repair possible damage, and enhance your inner and outer radiance—in short to make the most of this gift that was offered to us all called LIFE. You are a multileveled being, so I have included practices for your emotional body, your mental body, and, of course, your spirit. Any less would simply be too limiting and would take from your potential, which is infinite!

The information shared here covers the full spectrum of anti-aging tips and rejuvenating treatments, for men and women of all ages. Although this book is largely based on natural and simple practices, I have also included a research on cosmetic procedures because it is a fact that many people use all they can to look and feel better about themselves.

Why would you want to read this book?

And what could you possibly read here that you haven't already read somewhere else? Quite a lot, in fact; there is plenty of misleading information when it comes to anti-aging products and ways to improve your looks. It has become a massive industry. The people you would tend to ask for advice are those who are potentially selling you some kind of product or procedure, so their advice is often biased. Unfortunately, a lot of cosmetic products do not deliver on their promises—so you can often waste time and money *and* find that your problem is still there ... and growing!

Added to this, methods that are free are not usually revealed, as there is no profit to be made from them, which is why I call them "secrets." You will find them all included here. My intention in writing this book is to inform you as best I can on the *whole spectrum* of anti-aging related issues, and really give you simple and easy practices I have used on myself for years. In fact, the first three chapters could be considered as my own private journal. While you may choose to explore certain practices and not others, you will certainly have fun exploring or maybe simply remembering what you already know. Reference books from great authors on all the practices treated here are included, should you wish to deepen your studies. This book's mission is to bring clarity and information, so that your decisions are made in the light of knowledge and with increased awareness. The power is with you!

A stress-free life

Life *can be* easy, believe it or not! So the desire to live in health and beauty should not be a source of stress, pressure or guilt, as it often is. We all know that modern living provides us with plenty of these as it is. If you are one of those people who always try to do everything perfectly, NOW might be a good time to take a liberating breath and let it all go. Who is judging you, anyway? Only you, in a way that really matters, so take it easy on yourself! Why not start enjoying life and having a bit more fun, and yes, probably messing things up at times! I am a great believer in bringing moderation and awareness into *everything we do*. If you don't like some of the tips offered here, please do not try to convince yourself otherwise; your instinct is your guiding light: follow it. If, on the other hand, you choose to change a few of your habits, do it in your own time and have fun getting to know yourself better. You will be amazed and delighted at how good you feel, which will help to shift the way you perceive yourself physically; and you will begin to appreciate how beautiful you really are! Of course, as you radiate, this will be apparent to other people too, so don't be surprised if your friends and family ask to know your secrets!

You will also find some practical tips and exercises on how to stay or become aware throughout your daily life: this is the ultimate remedy for stress. Stress is one of the most aging factors and the root cause of many illnesses, so imagine being able to use a "safety rope" whenever you feel that you are drowning in the daily hustle and bustle. Not only will you start to enjoy life for what it is, but you will also benefit from major rejuvenation … guaranteed! Respecting your own body and living consciously naturally promotes living a beautiful and productive life, on all levels. A lot of what is explored in this manual is based on simplicity and originates from ancient wisdom, using resources already within you.

How do you contribute to your health?

What are your thoughts on aging? Do you still go on the assumption, based on what you have heard until now, that: "There is nothing I can do about it; it is going to happen anyway." This much is obvious; however *you do have a choice* on *how* you move through life and how to affect the *quality of your existence*. In order to appreciate the value of some of the secrets enclosed in this manual, we will explore two of the main factors that contribute to the quality of your health and beauty: *the biological aging process* and the *power that your thoughts and your conditioning have on your emotional and physical body.* Another well-known myth is that 'good' or 'bad' genes are hereditary: you might be positively shocked that this accounts for less than 10 percent of your overall health; the rest is up to you. There is a large body of evidence (study of epigenetic science) proving that percentage is even lower than that—so how about taking 100 percent responsibility for your health, your life, and, ultimately, your destiny?

From life insurance to prevention

Most of you have life insurance. While this may give you a sense of security, the nature of any kind of insurance preys on the possibility that things will go wrong. When they do go wrong, and the list of possibilities is long, you can cash in on the policy. It's not much good when you no longer have good health; only then do we realize that *health is wealth*! While I am not suggesting for a second that you should not insure yourself and your health, I propose that you develop an ability to use *preventative care,* which is a different kind of life insurance that I like to call *vivid self-awareness*. This one is free of charge; and it includes all the bonuses and dividends you need to start experiencing natural, free-flowing abundance.

Most accidents and illnesses come disguised into our life as wake-up calls ranging from mild to very serious, depending on how asleep or numb we really are. They materialize to warn us that we are not taking good care of ourselves, or simply to invite us to be more present. Wake-up calls also happen to conscious people, as there is always room for more alertness. The tips you will find enclosed in this manual will help you to maintain, or acquire, greater health and self-awareness—physically, emotionally, and mentally. I am suggesting that *prevention* is the best kind of personal insurance you will ever have; this is what I call *preventative care* in the form of *vivid self-awareness*. When you live an aware life, you are far more receptive and therefore more likely to detect early symptoms of disease, long before it takes over your life. On a more general note, being more aware means that you are able to respect yourself in a way that is conducive to your own health and live a more peaceful and productive life altogether.

Understanding the aging process

To put it very simply, every second, thousands of new cells are formed as they replicate after splitting from the original one. As the years go by, the new cells produced are a fraction less complete than the original and, little by little, aging begins. The state and health of your cells is determined by what you put into your body and how you feel, but most importantly, by what your thoughts are. We are just beginning to understand the magnitude of the impact that *thought-forms* have on our emotional and physical health, and ultimately, how we co-create our reality.

Let's get started!

Chapter One

BASIC REJUVENATING SECRETS

1. Food: The Kind That is Super-Yummy and Energizing—Enough Dieting!

YOUR ATTITUDE TOWARD FOOD

Why take on another diet when *you know* that it only works for a limited period of time? You know that, before long, you will probably be back to your old habits, with added guilt and despair. Apart from the fact that regular dieting can actually damage your health and shorten your life, it is also a huge restriction to impose upon yourself, yielding short-lived results and often promoting a sense of wasted emotion. So how about making some simple adjustments that you can sustain throughout your daily routine that are practical, long-lasting, reasonable, and tasty? Let us look at your eating habits.

What kind of eater are you?

Do you eat:

- To simply feed yourself?
- To cover unpleasant emotions?
- Past your hunger and into indulgence on a regular basis?
- Out of boredom?

Are you conscious of what you eat when you do? Or do you just pile the food down to stop the hungry feeling? Take a moment now to become aware of your eating habits.

In reality, food is meant as a *medicine* for the body

Knowing and accepting this fact alone can have a profound impact on how you treat yourself and what kind of food you put into your body. It may shift your eating habits altogether if you are truly ready for change.

There is no harm in having an occasional treat, the kind that gives you instant gratification with little or no nutrition; this is fine if you do it because you love the food and it is occasional.

If, however, you 'treat' yourself in large amounts and on a daily basis, I don't have to tell you that there is something amiss: *you already know that yourself.* You also probably beat up on yourself for having indulged, which makes matters considerably worse.

The first step is to *acknowledge* your food habit. You may be aware of the emotional issue that you are covering up. If you are not, it is okay to *simply be aware* that there is an issue that needs to be looked at. It is more about *being* than *doing*.

The second step is to *become present* each time that you find yourself reaching for more; this may be done without effort and without trying to willfully alter your habitual pattern. You may find that as you become more aware around your eating habit, your compulsions naturally decrease.

Awareness Around Cravings exercise

Simply observe yourself in action next time you feel cravings coming on.

- As you become aware of your craving, simply take a deep breath and observe the *seemingly* magnetic pull that your body feels toward the food. This is only an old pattern running through you.
- Feel the intensity in your hand, as it wants to reach forward

and grab. Keep observing, focus on your breathing, and relax your body. Realize that it is only an outmoded habit.
- Don't judge or evaluate; simply continue to witness what is taking place in yourself, in your mind, and in your emotions. By remaining as *the observer*, you allow a deeper place to open up in you: your true essence, *that* which is pure consciousness, *that* which is who you truly are, *that* which you come from.

The deeper part of you that is beyond thoughts and emotions, *the witness within*, is the place of awareness that is also known as consciousness. If you can observe your own feelings and reactions—and know that they are *in you* but cannot define you, as they are not really *who you truly are*—you are on the road to freedom from your negative habit. This may take a little time to establish, as you have been running on old habits for a number of years, so be gentle with yourself.

You ate it anyway?

That's okay; don't give yourself a hard time—enjoy it! Keep watching, being aware; this will change with repeated practice. Your willingness to change and your newfound awareness will ensure that results will be prompt and durable. To shift deeply ingrained and subconscious habits, have a look at my program at The Academy of Luminaries, where I transmit the Mahayana Method, a simple three step process used to eliminate all self-limitations; check out www.iagentofchange.com for more details. You might also find EFT (the emotional freedom technique) useful; check out www.eftuniverse.com for more details.

A NOTE ON WEIGHT LOSS

A large amount of the vocabulary used around weight loss pertains to reinforcing the issue at hand. If all you think about is losing weight—not eating too much, weighing yourself daily or several times a day—you are giving the issue all the attention it needs to grow!

Energy follows thoughts—so simply make up your mind about wanting to feel at home in your own body and living your very best life. Once your mind is made up, the "doing" becomes effortless. You will find that you naturally start to choose a style of nutrition that enhances and supports your decision. Gratitude plays a huge part in how you feel, so develop a sense of love and appreciation for your body, which is literally the temple of your soul and your vehicle to navigate this life.

A rule of thumb: balance is always a wise choice; so if you eat healthy and nutritious food 80 percent of the time, you can afford to relax and indulge a little the rest of the time, which is 20 percent. A pretty good deal, wouldn't you say?

Attitude around food

Are you vegetarian, vegan, macrobiotic; or do you simply eat a little of everything? It really doesn't matter right here, right now. I am not going to challenge your beliefs; but I do invite you to think about *your attitude* toward your food of choice. Whether you prefer a bowl of porridge and a smoothie or a large croissant with ham and melted cheese accompanied by a strong cup of coffee, the most important thing you can do is to enjoy it: eat it in peace and with awareness. It'll taste a whole lot better.

To a certain extent, the *judgment* you put upon yourself affects you as much as (if not more than) as the kind of food you eat, so relax and delight in your meal! Love your food, it will love you back. Become aware of *how you eat* your food and *what your thoughts and feelings* are while you do so. Know that you absorb whatever emotions you feel while you eat; so if you are angry or upset, wait until you feel better. The last thing you want to eat is toasted rage or guilt.

REFINED FOOD

Refined food is best avoided altogether

This includes all the white stuff available in most food stores. It is food that has literally been bleached, leaving little or no nutrients in it. During the First World War, white bread was considered to be more "classy" than the brown variety because of a lack of information, but we now know that this is not the case. We understand that most vitamins, fiber, and vital nutrients remain if the food has been processed as little as possible. The choice is yours.

Commonly used bleached products include:

White bread
White rice
White pasta
White flour
White salt
Anything bright white, basically!

Tip: Why not start by replacing one refined product with a whole meal variety each week? This may regulate your bowels movements if you are constipated.

WHEN IS THE BEST TIME TO EAT?

Stating the obvious: but eating is best when hungry *only*!

There have been plenty of times when you and I have eaten without being hungry. This not only wastes food but also a large amount of your energy that is taken up by digestion. Most of us need food every four hours; of course, this depends on the individual. Some people may prefer smaller meals more frequently, which is absolutely fine.

The golden rule, however, is to leave a gap of two or three hours between the last meal and your bedtime. Otherwise, food just sits in the stomach more or less undigested overnight, leaving the body feeling full and bloated on rising. You will find that sleep is more peaceful and rejuvenating if your body has had a chance to "wind down" before resting.

Tips: These may sound obvious but are unfortunately often ignored.

- *Stop eating before you feel full.* Let the food settle after your last helping, you might find that you are satisfied without reaching for more.
- Adequate *chewing* is essential as it breaks down the nutrients and mixes them with saliva, which contains important enzymes to assist the digestive process. Try chewing your mouthful a minimum of twenty times for best results.

ORGANIC FOOD

Treat yourself … you are *definitely* worth it!

How much organic food do you buy? Today, organic produce is widely available and, as more people choose this natural option, it is becoming more accessible to us all, both practically and financially; and it is a significant contribution to personal and planetary global health. Even if you only buy a few organic things each week, you are doing yourself a great favor. You might like to prioritize buying fruits and vegetables that you can eat without peeling off the skin. Why? Because the amount of spray used on the produce can have such a polluting impact on your health that these items are simply not worth eating.

Tip: For non-organic produce, add a little cider vinegar to the rinsing water. This will help in removing pesticides and some of the other chemicals that have been sprayed onto the food.

Meat and fish are better eaten less often, and from wild or organic origin *only.*

Eating animal protein everyday is not necessary for good health—quite the contrary. Fresh fish and/or meat eaten two to three times per week is perfectly acceptable from a health point of view. I was born in France, where it is common practice to eat meat twice a day, which would be served after a starter of cold salted meat such as ham and *saucisson.* This is probably why the French are known to "dig their tombs with their teeth!"

It is particularly important to choose organic produce, or at the very least free-range, when it comes to buying fish and meat. Mass-produced nonorganic meat and fish is excessively treated for speedy growth and larger profit, and to avoid the proliferation of diseases due to poor sanitary conditions and reduced living space. Eating a battery-caged chicken, turkey, or any other unfortunate animal that never had the experience of fresh air and green fields can be a sad and disturbing experience. It means eating MISERY. Could this be a contributing factor to the depressed feeling that most people experience after Thanksgiving or Christmas dinner?

ON ALLERGIES

Have you noticed that so many people are allergic to so many things nowadays? Maybe you are suffering some kind of allergy yourself? There is a very good possibility that it isn't the food you or they are allergic to, but rather the fertilizers, pesticides, growth boosters, or other drugs injected into it.

Tip: If you suffer from food intolerances and would like to know more about this, look for a reputable kinesiologist in your area. A kinesiologist uses a simple muscle reflex technique that identifies the allergies and their origin, and can also offer guidelines for correcting imbalances. The problem could originate from living or working in a toxic environment, whether it is due to physical, electrical, or emotional stress. It could be a simple reaction to something such as: household products, neon lighting, makeup, food fertilizer, or… possibly your present choice of employment!

For example:

—Let's say that you seem to be allergic to broccoli. It would be a good idea to be tested with one piece of broccoli that is organic and one that isn't. This will accurately point to the origin of the allergy. It would be a shame to dismiss certain produce altogether because of the inaccuracy of the source of stress.

—At the office, it might be the lighting that causes you to experience those migraines, or the long hours of staring at the computer screen rather than your coworker or boss as you thought! See pages 34 & 228 for tips on the use of crystals to help eliminate electrical stress.

GRAINS ARE NOT JUST FOR THE BIRDS!

Whole grains are the most obvious types of food that are lacking in Western diets

This is a shame because but they are a wonderful food, full of essential nutrients. In fact *you could survive on them alone!* So including some whole grain in your diet would be a valuable gift to your health. Grains are super-nutritious with a rich portfolio of protein and amino acids, making them a fantastic food for everyone and especially important for those of you who are vegetarian or vegan (an absolute "must" if you are pregnant and living such a lifestyle). Whole grains are full of vitamins and they keep the blood-sugar levels very stable, making them a great asset for busy people who require a high level of mental and physical performance. They're also great for anyone studying and taking exams—kids and grownups alike. If you are prone to PMS (pre-menstrual syndrome) and usually experience symptoms such as crazy mood swings, you may find that eating millet prior to that particular week has a balancing effect. This grain is generally nurturing for the whole female reproductive system.

Most whole grains are available in all health food stores and can also be found in supermarkets. Whole grains are easy to cook but can taste quite bland for the most part, so they can be mixed with sauces, fruits, vegetables, or spices. They are very versatile.

List of whole grains:

Amaranth
Millet
Bulgur
Barley
Buckwheat
Couscous (wholemeal)
Quinoa
Rye
All brown rice (basmati, risotto, etc.)
Spelt

If you would like to see a considerable improvement in your health and vitality, include a helping of whole grain in your daily menu. You will notice the benefit on your skin almost immediately as it regains its lustrous appearance. A lot of very beautiful and seemingly ageless ethnicities such as Chinese, African and Indian, have had the wisdom to eat whole grains for centuries and have benefited from its gift of health and longevity since the dawn of civilization.

Millet: Records show that it is the oldest grain known to mankind and was already eaten by our ancestors, the Egyptians. In the realm of whole grains, quite a few qualify as super-foods, but millet is undoubtedly "the King," as described by Dr. Paavo Airola in his book, *Worldwide Secrets for Staying Young* (see Bibliography). It is one of the most nutritious grains, with an impressive portfolio of B vitamins, calcium, potassium, iron, zinc, and magnesium. It contains no gluten, making it suitable for people with wheat intolerance (celiac disease). It is the *only grain* that is alkaline once ingested (see pages 11-13 for acid/alkali food information).

Quinoa: This is the next best whole grain, also suitable for celiacs. It has a balanced set of amino acids, making it another complete nutrient in itself.

Note: I agree with you that making a sandwich with grains is virtually impossible! This undoubtedly means that you may have to invest ten minutes in boiling some whole grain of your choice. Think of the amount of time you give to a cause or other people each day and realize that you deserve no less yourself ... there is only one of you! Whole grain is full of natural fiber, which promotes regular bowel movement. Fiber taken in this form does not irritate the stomach lining, as bran or laxatives can do. Another incentive is that a regular bowel ensures that your skin glows!

Tip 1: If you would like to make an easy switch from bread to whole grain, why not boil a little millet, quinoa, or brown rice and leave it to cool down overnight. It can be added to your salads or eaten alongside a soup. Try sprinkling some soy sauce into it for extra flavor. This can be taken literally anywhere: to the office, in your car, or at break times.

Tip 2: If you don't feel ready to start using whole grains just yet, why not choose to buy whole-grain bread instead? There is a lot of good homemade bread available in most shops nowadays, so you can stay away from sliced pan very easily! Have you tried spelt or rye bread? It makes a welcome change from eating an overload of wheat products, which is often the cause of allergies and constipation.

Easy ways to use whole grains

This is for millet, quinoa, or any other wholegrain of your choice:

- Simply boil your grain in slightly salted water for about ten or fifteen minutes or until it is soft enough to eat.
- Serve it for breakfast as a sweet dish with honey, sugar, raisins, or dates.
- Eat it as a savory meal with salt, soy sauce, tomato sauce, olive oil, or a few steamed vegetables.
- Eat it cold, as an added ingredient or made into a salad (think tabouli!); it can be taken virtually anywhere.
- Use it to replace the usual potatoes when eating a fish or meat dish and to add variety to any main courses at home.

ACID- AND ALKALINE-FORMING FOODS

Acid and alkaline balance in the body

The pH scale ranges from 0 to 14. Any foods with numbers below 7 are considered acid and, therefore, low in oxygen; anything numbered above 7 is alkaline and oxygen-rich. Healthy blood has a pH of 7.4, which inhibits the development of cancer cells, and blood with a pH above 8.5 eradicates the presence of any diseased cells in the body.

To maintain optimum health, your diet should include 60

percent of alkalizing foods and 40 percent of acid-forming foods. If you need to restore balance in your diet, you can eat 80 percent alkalizing foods and only 20 percent acid-forming for a while. Food contains both acid and alkaline qualities before they are ingested, and are either acid- or alkaline-forming once digested. In general, natural foods are alkaline-forming while manufactured and processed foods are acid forming. A large intake of acid-forming foods can contribute to the development of diseases, ranging from mild to very serious, and of course, it accelerates the aging process.

If there is too much acidity in the body:

- The risk of fatigue and illness is greatly increased.
- The absorption of vital minerals and nutrients is decreased.
- There is a toxic overload and a reduced ability to deal with elimination.
- The cells are deprived of oxygen and their production is decreased.

In our Western diets, acidity is prevalent as too much animal protein and dairy are consumed on a daily basis. Large amounts of alcohol, fried foods, and chemical food substitutes, such as artificial sweeteners, contribute to an overload of acidity in the body.

On a more general note, people who suffer regular indigestion, who are prone to ailments such as arthritis and rheumatism, sufferers of migraines, constipation, etc., would benefit enormously from introducing more alkalizing foods in their diets.

Acid-forming foods:

All dairies (with the exception of goat milk and cheese)
Fish and meat
Most whole grains
All fried foods

Alcohol, tea, and coffee
Medicinal and recreational drugs
Most nuts
Breads and cakes
Olives and pickles
Plums and prunes
Blueberries and cranberries
Corn and lentils

I know what you are thinking … is there anything left to eat?! Yes there is some good food included in the following category.

Alkaline-forming foods:
Nearly all fruits and vegetables (except those named above)
Almonds
Tofu and tempeh (found in health food stores)
Apple cider vinegar
Probiotic cultures and soured dairies
Fresh fruit and vegetable juices
Millet
Herbal teas
Flax, sunflower, and pumpkin seeds
All herbs
Dried dates and figs
Sauerkraut
Seaweed

Tip: Again, be gentle on yourself and start by increasing your intake of fruits and vegetables. If you know you are going to have a very acidic meal, a glass of carrot juice taken with the meal has an alkalinizing effect on the digestive system. Digestive enzymes also help with difficult digestion and can be bought in any good health food store.

WHAT ABOUT CEREALS?

BREAK-FAST means that you are breaking the overnight fast

So choosing what to put in your body first thing in the morning is important. It is a well-known fact that there is absolutely *nothing good* in most commercial cereals. They are laced with all types of sugars, which give the body a 'high' for about half an hour before taxing vital energy for the rest of the morning. Hunger surfaces rapidly, and staying focused until lunchtime is nearly impossible. Not particularly helpful for students or anyone else who has to perform using their optimal concentration throughout the morning (e.g., meetings, presentations, studies).

General tip: On rising, a large glass of water half an hour before any food is taken is extremely beneficial, as it rehydrates the system. This can be cold, warm, or hot water. Adding half of a freshly squeezed lemon makes this a liver-tonic, which is beneficial for all, particularly for those who have had a few glasses of alcohol the previous night.

Healthy breakfast ideas

- Smoothies are great, especially those made with probiotic yogurt or kefir (a fermented milk drink available in Eastern European grocery stores). Smoothies are also great without any dairy. Soy or rice milk can be used for people with lactose intolerance. Some whole-grain bread with nut butter or jam can be added if you still feel hungry.
- A bowl of millet (you can buy millet flakes in most health food stores) or oat porridge is really great for keeping hunger at bay all morning long.
- Remember that you can simply boil some grain and add your favorite ingredients to it: dates, raisin, figs, etc.

WHAT ABOUT SALT?

Are you one of those salt addicts?

Do you always add salt without tasting the food first? You probably already know that you are increasing your chances of heart disease each time you reach out for more? A large amount of salt eaten on a daily basis can contribute to the narrowing of your arteries, which in turns reduces your heart's ability to function properly, so re-educating your taste buds is vital!

I would like to invite you to *become conscious* the moment you reach for the salt dispenser. Why not try the food that is served to you before automatically adding salt to it? Examine the origin of the belief you hold when you say: "Oh, it's just a habit I have—I can't do anything about it." Sure you can! I have a higher opinion of you; I firmly believe that you are strong enough to get a handle on your salt intake to modify its quantity and quality if and when *you choose to.* This may take a little while, as you need to retrain your body to taste the food without the usual overload of salt. Or maybe you can make up your mind easily and change spontaneously. You might find that having the *willpower* to make your own decisions based on the *quality of your health* is ultimately more self-empowering than falling prey to old habits that don't serve you in any way.

Some amount of salt, however, is vital for good health

The kind of salt you use is important, as some salt is better than others. You may have guessed it by now: the refined white kind that most people use is not so good at all, while the unrefined variety is in fact more beneficial, if used in moderation, as always. You may first need to take a closer look at what you eat; how much and what kind of salt you are absorbing:

- If you are a lover of junk food and eat it regularly, you probably have too much salt in your system already, and not of the good kind.
- If you only eat the *occasional* chips, snacks, or other

processed foods, you might be okay, but make sure you start using unrefined salt at home.

- If you cook most of the food you eat, you have a direct choice as to what kind of salt and how much you use, so this is the best situation!

Tip: Use unrefined salt only. This salt is pale gray because it hasn't been bleached and, therefore, isn't completely stripped of all its natural goodness. There are no anti-caking agents in it either, so you may have to rub it between your fingertips to thin it out a little before use … no big deal! It contains around seventy-five essential minerals that your body needs—which is great—as vitamins and minerals from a natural source are always more readily absorbable than those in vitamin pills.

WHAT ABOUT SUGAR?

We all love it!

Sugar is the tastiest, most readily available addictive "drug" you can find anywhere. Available to rich and poor, young and old, it is hidden in nearly all man-made foodstuffs and in everything that is precooked (along with its twin, salt). There is nothing positive to say about the addition to sugar in your diet. It wears many different forms and names, which makes it hard to identify.

Here are some of its different names:

Glucose
Lactose
Dextrose
Malt
Fructose
Maple syrup
Corn syrup

Molasses
Syrup
Brown sugar
Treacle
Honey
Caramel
Sugar cane
Most commercial cereals often have three or four of the above.

Note of caution on artificial sweeteners

Having said all that, if you want to eat something sweet, do yourself a *guilt-free favor* and have some real sugar! Don't think that having a synthetic replacement is better for your health; it isn't. Some research points out that artificial sweeteners may in fact contribute to the detriment of your health and, in some cases, to cancer. If you want to replace sugar, you can use honey, date syrup, or *real* maple syrup. They all contain powerful nutrients and vitamins and are exquisitely sweet. Reducing your sugar intake altogether would be better still, particularly if you want to shed some weight and keep your youthful looks.

Tip: Try cooking your porridge with dates (or another dry fruit of your choice) for a change; it is delicious and really good for you. Dates are naturally very sweet and packed with plenty of fiber, vitamins, and minerals (notably iron). They soften while the porridge is cooking, making it sweet and creamy and eliminating the need to add sugar or honey. Yum!

Note: I understand that coffee wouldn't have the same appeal with a date lying at the bottom of your cup, so, as always: there is no harm in an occasional treat.

Moderation is the mother of good health!

THE MIRACULOUS SPROUTING SEEDS

How to perform a small health miracle for yourself

Sprouting seeds is extremely easy, and the benefits of eating them are *enormous*. That's right; those little seeds are nothing short of miraculous! Some supermarkets sell them sprouted, although they can become soggy and lose their precious nutrients quite fast while stored in the bright light on the shelves. To be honest, sprouts are so quick and easy to grow that they are actually not worth buying, even if you are really busy. If I can do it, you can do it! And consider this: *a handful of sprouted seeds contains as much vitamins, minerals, and enzymes as a regular serving of vegetables*. Wow!

List of some seeds you can sprout:

Alfalfa
Broccoli
Lentil
Mung bean
Quinoa
Radish
Red clover (helpful for men and women as it contains protective qualities for the prostate gland, and also has plant hormones for women in need of help while enduring PMT [pre-menstrual tension], or going through menopause)
Fenugreek
Mustard seeds

Most of them are high in vitamins A, B, C, and E, as well as minerals and trace elements that the body needs. They are handy to carry around in your lunch box, when in the office or while traveling. They make a tasty addition, topping your salads or sandwiches (instead of limp lettuce leaves) or sprinkled over any dishes at home. You don't need a sprouter (unless you really want to buy one) or any other fancy equipment: just seeds. *Organic is a must,* as others will probably have been genetically modified and will therefore not be as nutritious.

Sprouting made easy

1. Soak your chosen seeds in a little bowl of water for about twelve hours, starting with a small amount, like a soupspoon.
2. The next day, drain them (a tea strainer does the trick) and leave them on your windowsill. Cover the dish with a little piece of muslin or any other material thin enough to let the seeds "breathe"; otherwise they will mold.
3. Rinse and drain them twice a day (morning and night) until they grow two or three inches in height.

Soon enough, and depending on the room temperature and the time of the year, those seeds will grow into sprouts—within three to five days. You are growing your very own super-food!

Tip 1: When they are about an inch tall, let them grow for another couple of days without covering them up with muslin; the tops will become bright green, charged with chlorophyll: another precious super-food. Chlorophyll can help to rejuvenate the liver, has antibacterial properties, and acts as a wound healer. It also has anti-inflammatory properties for those people who have arthritis and suffer from skin complaints. It is also a much sought-after antioxidant said to prevent the signs of aging. Both chlorophyll and various other antioxidants can be purchased in health food stores at quite a substantial price. While I am not against supplements at all, if the food eaten can provide most of the vitamins and minerals needed by the body and is extracted more efficiently, why not use it? It is money saved in your pocket, health and vitality stored in your body!

Tip 2: Keep your sprouted seeds in a closed container in the fridge, and eat them within two or three days so they are crisp and full of the promised wonders.

MORE HEALTHY SEEDS

We are blessed with many other great seeds

There are plenty of other types of seeds that are also packed with vitamins, fiber, and rejuvenating properties. They're very handy while traveling or at work in place of a snack for an emergency energy boost!

Delicious seeds include:

Linseed (same as flaxseed)
Hemp seeds
Poppy seeds
Pumpkin seeds
Sesame seeds
Sunflower seeds

The following make tasty snacks and are particularly beautifying:

Sesame seeds have a very distinctive nutty flavor and are used in a wide variety of confectionary sweets, breads, and notably on top of burger buns, where they usually sit sadly bleached to death! Choose the unbleached seeds for top nutrition. A pleasant way to eat sesame seeds is using tahini, which is made from the pulp of sesame seeds. It tastes delicious and is packed with good oils: a real treat for your health and your skin. It is richer in calcium than cheese, milk, and even nuts. It contains essential fatty acids (EFAs), plenty of vitamin E, B6, and B12; copper; manganese; and zinc. You may already be familiar with "halvah," which is a deliciously sweet confectionary originating from the Middle East and made from tahini. Traditional hummus is also made with tahini.

Tip: Try mixing some tahini with some honey for a delicious and healthy snack/dessert. The proportion of honey very much depends on how sweet you like it. Why not use Manuka honey (from New Zealand; said to have antibacterial properties) if you want to make it a particularly potent and healing snack? Put the leftover mixture (if you've managed not to eat it all) in the fridge—it becomes like a rich fudge!

Pumpkin seeds are beneficial for us all, but particularly for younger men going through puberty, and more mature men who wish to keep their prostate gland in optimal health. These seeds contain many of the B vitamins, calcium, iron, magnesium, phosphorus, potassium, zinc and are said to be beneficial for the prevention of depression.

Sunflower seeds are packed with the same goodness as the pumpkin seeds, but have superior levels of vitamin E, making them a wonderful food for the elasticity and suppleness of the skin. They are also notably high in iron.

Delicious TV snack

Here is a very healthy, easy to make, and incredibly tasty TV snack that the whole family will love. It is a great alternative to chips for any kind of festive occasion.

1. Dry roast pumpkin and sunflower seeds in a pan for a few seconds *only*; this will ensure that they do not lose all their good oils.
2. Before you take the pan off the stove, throw a dash of soy sauce onto the seeds (tamari is delicious); it will sizzle madly so mix them around quickly for one or two seconds.
3. Pour the seeds into a little dish.

They're ready to eat and absolutely scrumptious!

LET'S GO NUTS!

Nuts are super-nutritious and their gift to you is an impressive portfolio of vitamins and minerals

Do stay away from eating too much of the salted variety for obvious reasons (see section on salt, page **15**). They make a wonderful and handy snack whether at the office, while traveling, or at home. They are lovely added to a stir-fry or salad, and of course in cakes and pastries. Although all nuts are good for your health, only almonds and chestnuts are alkalizing to the digestive system. A handful of nuts a day is great; they are rich in oils, so any more than that is only good if you are trying to put on weight.

List of scrumptious nuts:

Almond
Peanuts
Chestnuts
Pecan nuts
Brazil nuts
Pine nuts
Cashew nuts
Pistachios
Hazelnuts
Walnuts
Macadamia nuts

Wonderful almonds

Eating almonds is said to be very beneficial in lowering bad cholesterol while providing the body with ample amounts of vitamin E. Vitamin E promotes good blood circulation and keeps the arteries supple, so they help your heart to keep beating with youth and vitality. Almonds are very filling and packed with fiber, so they also contribute to regular and healthy bowel habits.

Tip: For a super-beautifying and exceptionally nutritious treat, try *sprouted almonds*. Soak a handful of almonds in water overnight, in the same way you started to sprout seeds. In the morning, strain them and put them on a towel; pat them dry and store them in your fridge. They taste very "green," as they have effectively regained their freshness and a few hundred percent of vitamins ... all your cells will vibrate with pleasure!

WHY ARE ANTIOXIDANTS SO FASHIONABLE?

Antioxidants are powerful natural plant elements that fight free radicals and protect your body.

Okay, so what are free radicals?

Free radicals are highly reactive molecules capable of causing serious damage to the brain and other vital cellular molecules such as DNA, speeding up the *aging process* on tissues and organs, and causing many diseases to proliferate.

Free radicals are produced when:

- You inhale smoke (of any kind)
- You live in a polluted area
- You eat fried food and "bad" fats
- You absorb an overload of toxins
- You take too much sunlight or go through radiation therapy
- You are under severe stress

Antioxidants: Fruits and vegetables are your best friends!

Antioxidants prevent the oxidation of your cells and are therefore helpful in preventing and repairing the damage caused by free radicals. Antioxidants protect your arteries from hardening, thereby keeping heart problems, premature aging, Alzheimer's disease, cancer, and many more serious problems at bay. This is why antioxidants are so fashionable nowadays. It is also a great idea to eat as many different colors and variety of fruits and vegetables as possible every day; they all have different and necessary vital properties. They are full of fiber and precious life-sustaining moisture. A large amount of the vegetables you eat are best eaten raw every day, as many enzymes are destroyed when cooked. The contrary is true for certain vegetables, such as tomatoes, which have added benefits when cooked: lycopene is released and is known to be a powerful antioxidant that contributes to the prevention and healing of certain cancers, notably of the prostate. You have also probably come across facial beauty cosmetics with lycopene, as it wonderful for promoting glowing skin.

Tip: Why not cook up a delicious red sauce to go with some whole-meal pasta using organic produce? Accompanied by a glass of good-quality red wine, this makes a wonderfully healthy and rejuvenating treat!

Juices: An easy way to consume your daily raw antioxidants

There are all kinds of wonderful juices and smoothies available to buy ready-made if you are under pressure in the morning. Even better: why not invest in a juicer or/and a blender to make your own mixtures at home? Fresh juices are also discussed on pages 149-151.

The following exotic fruits make absolutely gorgeous smoothies packed full of vitamins, cleansing out the system; and all have amazing health- and beauty-boosting properties:

Papaya and mango
Lychees and pineapple
Guava and coconut
Passion fruit
Berries (all types)
Banana

Note: Orange juice is fine, but it can be very acidic and hard to digest for people with a fragile stomach. You may also be citrus–intolerant, and it can be hard to find a commercial juice that does not contain oranges. In this case, buying a juicer is a very smart investment that will give you regular health dividends forever!

Powerful super-antioxidant fruits:

Blueberries
Cranberries
Blackberries
Blackcurrants
Juniper berries (they add a great taste to sauerkraut)
Pomegranate (available as a juice extract in health food stores)
Red grapes
Cherries, prunes, and apricots
Umeboshi plums
Acai berries
Goji berries
Dates
Figs

Do you remember your mother telling you to eat your greens?

She was right and you know it! All the dark leafy vegetables (cabbage, spinach, watercress, rocket, etc.), all the dark-colored root vegetables (carrots, beetroot, etc.), literally *all vegetables* are really good for you, and they can be really fun to cook too. They all contain various vitamins such as A and C, iron, beta-carotene, and plenty of minerals and phytonutrients.

The one drawback about "regular meat eaters" is that, in their diet, vegetables are not always utilized to their full potential. Most of the creativity goes into the meat or fish dish, leaving the poor lonely vegetables on the side as garnish … what a shame! Try buying some vegetarian or vegan cook books to broaden your horizons on cooking with vegetables, beans, grains, seeds, and nuts—and have fun in the kitchen trying new things! Eva Batt, in her book *Vegan Cooking* (5), shares many innovative and tasty recipes. You'll be amazed at what delicious novelties you can cook up! Kids love having fun too, and if they have contributed to making a mealtime dish, I bet you anything that you'll be able to get them eat it, no matter how green it is! The benefits of good nutrition are endless, and remember, since we are talking about looking good and feeling fantastic here, it would be sad to not take advantage of Mother Nature's abundant gifts! There are also plenty of antioxidants in herbs and vitamins, which we will look at on pages 44 & 61. Here is one of my favorite recipes:

Rejuvenating cabbage stir-fry recipe

For this beautifying and health-boosting recipe, you'll need:

One-half an organic curly (or any) cabbage
One soupspoon of extra-virgin olive oil
One onion
One handful of pine nuts
One handful of feta cheese cubes
One dash of soy sauce or pinch of salt
Black pepper to taste

In a wok or frying pan

Heat the soupspoon of olive oil.

Add the onion, *chopped,* the pinch of unrefined salt (or soy sauce), and the handful of pine nuts.

Let this fry for three or four minutes, and then add:

The one-half curly cabbage, *chopped.*

Fry for just a few minutes, so the cabbage is still bright green and crunchy.

At the last moment add:

A handful of feta cheese cubes. Mix and serve up immediately. Add freshly ground pepper to taste.

Bon appétit!

Tip: Keeping a "food diary" can be a great way to monitor what you eat and what reacts with your digestive system. It can also give you an incentive to go for a walk when you look back and see that you over-indulged the day before. It works for me!

Naughty treats full of antioxidants

These two definitely feature in my diet anyway!

- Dark chocolate (minimum 70 percent cocoa)
- Red wine (good-quality)

Again, moderation plays a big role here. A few squares of chocolate satisfy the cravings for desserts or sweets and happen to be full of antioxidants, potassium, and magnesium. It may be an acquired taste, but it is definitely worth giving it a go. If you get to like it, you won't be able to eat the other types of chocolate, as once you make the switch you will realize that they are sickly sweet! Regarding the wine, I am talking about one glass a day, with your meal. At that rate, you can afford a good bottle, so have a little fun trying different types of wines that you might like. Wine cuts through grease: if you are a meat eater, it is a very valuable addition to your list of rejuvenating drinks.

Anti-Aging proverb!

A few squares of dark chocolate and a glass of red wine a day keep the doctor away!

TOPICS EXPLORED IN SECTION 1

- What is your attitude toward the food you eat?
- Awareness Around Cravings exercise
- When do you eat?
- What kind of food do you eat?
- Do you eat any whole grains?
- Do you have a balanced acid/alkaline diet?
- How much salt and sugar do you eat?
- Do you use sprouting seeds, nuts?
- How many fruits and vegetables do you eat, raw and cooked?

NOTES

2. Water and Its Benefits

DO YOU REALLY HAVE TO DRINK WATER?

We lose between three and five liters of water over a twenty-four-hour period

This takes places via our breath, perspiration, and urine, so yes: drinking water would be a good idea. How much? Again, it depends on your lifestyle. There are many different opinions on the subject, so let us use our common sense and learn or remember the simple biological facts about our body. We are made up of about 75 percent water; only 25 percent of our body is solid matter. If you exercise a lot, you need to drink more, as you are producing more sweat. In general, drinking between 1 and 1.5 liters should be fine. Always check how you feel; you may need more, or you may need less. Some people report ill effects from drinking too much water. There is no point following any kind of advice blindly or ignoring *how you feel;* be sensitive to you own signals and respect your own "feel-o-meter"! Being in tune with your own rhythms is far more important than following anybody's advice.

Some fruit and vegetable juice should also be consumed, fresh whenever possible. If you eat plenty of fresh fruits and vegetables every day and drink a minimum of 1.5 liters of water a day, you are absorbing plenty of wonderful moisture.

CAN YOU DRINK TEA, COFFEE, OR FIZZY DRINKS INSTEAD OF WATER?

Regular tea and coffee are both diuretics, which dehydrate the body So, I'm sorry to say that the answer is no. You still have to drink some water. Have you ever noticed that you urinate far more liquid than you have taken in after a cup of regular tea or coffee?

Not all teas are bad, however; see page 61 for more information. In fact, coffee has positive qualities, as it is packed with antioxidants. It was originally used in Brazil as a natural tonic for people with low blood pressure; but again, moderation is the key here. There is no harm in enjoying a cup of coffee or tea once or twice a day if that pleases you. Just make sure you drink an extra glass of water with every cup to rehydrate your system.

Fizzy drinks do absolutely nothing positive for you

Fizzy drinks are laced with sugar or, even worse, with artificial sweeteners; they do nothing to quench your thirst and give you extra calories you don't need. In fact, if you are trying to lose weight, simply cutting out fizzy drinks will give you a huge head start. Cordials are also sugar-laden. Good-quality fruit juice is great once or twice a day; just check the label to see that no extra sugar has been added, as fruit usually is sweet enough on its own.

BEAUTIFUL SKIN

Beautiful skin, soft and glowing, shows up when the body is free from toxic waste

The skin is the largest excretory system in the body—not the bowels, as commonly thought. This is why people who suffer from chronic constipation or do no physical activities can have dry, lifeless skin. The body never lies. Constipation can be the root cause of many health issues, such as apathy, depression, bad breath, prostate and colon cancer, enlargement of the colon, etc. It feels really awful to carry all that waste around all day and take it to bed each night. If someone handed you a bag of your own waste, you would run a mile! *There are no creams you can buy or any beautifying treatments you can have that will cover up overloaded skin.*

Drinking more water will certainly contribute toward the

elimination of constipation and replenish fluids lost through sweating while exercising. More whole grains, fruits, and vegetables should be eaten every day. Refined products must be *completely* eliminated if the problem is chronic. See page **66** for more information on alleviating constipation.

Tip 1: A pint of water (warm is more effective) taken on rising can really help the bowels to move. Add some freshly squeezed organic lemon juice to freshen up the breath and provide a generous amount of natural vitamin C to start the day.

Tip 2: A glass of prune juice can be taken first thing in the morning or any time during the day to promote healthy bowel movements. Prunes are powerful antioxidants and they are packed full of fiber—a really good friend to have nearby at anytime!

WILL THERE BE TIME TO DRINK ALL THAT WATER?

Absolutely! Drinking water is a positive habit you can adopt in no time once you have made your decision

Make sure you have a bottle with you at the office, in your car, and even at home to keep track of how much you are drinking. The best time to drink water is *between meals,* which is perfect, as it will help reduce or even satisfy the desire for snacking.

Water can be taken with meals but should be kept to a minimum, as it dilutes gastric juices necessary for good digestion. A large glass of water taken thirty minutes before a meal will suppress your appetite.

Example: A client of mine once said that she absolutely could not swallow a single mouthful of food without a big sip of water to wash down each bite. She was carrying unwanted weight and her skin lacked luster. I explained to her that unless food is chewed thoroughly, it isn't digested efficiently; the digestive system has trouble extracting vital nutrients because of the lack of enzymes found in saliva. She started to take her time to chew her food and consequently found that she ate a lot less than usual and enjoyed the food more. Her digestion-related problems, such as uncomfortable bloating, indigestion, and heartburn, also disappeared.

If you are desperately thirsty at meal times, check:

- Is the food is too salty,
- Too spicy, or
- Too sweet
- Is this the only time you think about drinking water?

Note: Cravings between meals are often a simple need for more hydration.

Tip: Wait for about two hours or more to resume your water intake. This is because the body is still busy processing the food that you have just eaten, and gastric juices are best left undiluted to do their work for effective digestion and maximum absorption. If you have had a heavily salted meal, you will notice that you get incredibly thirsty soon after your meal; in that case, choose water instead of a fizzy drink.

Herbal recipe for indigestion

Indigestion or heartburn is easily remedied with a tincture of chamomile.

- Simply make a regular cup of chamomile herbal tea; the only difference is that you use two tea bags instead of one.
- Let it steep for about ten minutes, so the brew becomes very concentrated and acts as an herbal remedy.
- Drink it as hot as possible.

- Try not to use any sugar of any kind or honey, as are they are both acid-forming, which may very well be the cause of your discomfort in the first place.

See the Tummy-Rubbing exercise on pages 109-110.

DEHYDRATION, WHO CARES?

Important facts

I have been appealing to your vanity most of the time so far; however, some research suggests that dehydration can have devastating on the body all-around and that it *doesn't necessarily materialize as thirst*. Let us not forget that the brain, our most important asset, is 85 percent water. Some research has been done showing that prolonged dehydration can contribute to Alzheimer's disease, among other illnesses, such as cancer, AIDS, heart failure, obesity, cholesterol formation, etc.

Do a little research for yourself if you still think that you don't need to drink water. Dr. F. Batmanghelidj has written a most informative book called *Water for Health* (5), which I highly recommend, as it is very enlightening.

THE WATER CONTROVERSY

The best and easiest water to drink might just be from the tap.

What you hear about water can be mind-boggling! There is no need to rush out and buy liters of mineral water from the supermarket: it has been sitting in plastic, which means that plastic molecules are in the water, particularly if the bottle was left in a warm environment (delivery trucks and your car). So what to do? Unless you have a well (and even if you do, you should have your water checked regularly, particularly if you live around a farm that utilizes chemicals and fertilizers), the best and easiest water to drink might just be from your tap. That can sound a little outrageous, I know, especially for those of you who have been convinced to use bottled or filtered water. Some readily available commercial filters filter *everything* out of the water, including the minerals, which is not great either. If you are in any doubt about the safety of your tap water, simply have it tested. Again, let your common sense dictate the best course of action to follow.

Tip: If there is a temporary danger of waste residue present in the water, simply boil it and let it cool down. Filtering it would not get rid of all the waste anyway.

For everyday use, fill a large pottery or glass jug and cover it with a clean cotton cloth. If you wait just thirty minutes, the chlorine evaporates naturally, taking away that ghastly taste. Water should basically taste of *nothing*, and be pleasantly bland.

Re-energizing your tap water

Put a small, clear quartz, crystal in your water jug to charge up the water with wonderful healing and regenerative properties. Rinse the crystal whenever you wash the jug. A small piece of quartz crystal costs practically nothing and has powerful rejuvenating qualities. For more information on the healing properties of crystals, read *Crystals Co-Creators* (27) by Dorothy Roeder.

For absolutely innovative and groundbreaking information, see experiments conducted by Dr. Masaru Emoto on water and how you can energize it by simply sending it pure unconditional love! He explains that any water from any big city can be once again brought back to its pristine healing origins if it is sent the right kind of energy; check out www.life-enthusiast.com/twilight/research_emoto.htm for free videos on this.

Fun experiment

Animals are sensitive to energy. If you give a dog the choice between a bowl of regular tap water and a bowl of crystal water, it will drink from the latter. Animals perceive energy clearly and listen to their instinct … all admirable qualities!

See Chapter Four for more information on the use of crystals.

TOPICS EXPLORED IN SECTION 2

- How much water do you drink every day?
- Are you satisfied with your elimination?
- How many teas, coffees, and fizzy drinks do you consume?
- Including water-drinking in your daily routine

NOTES

3. Beauty Products You Can Find in Your Kitchen

FOODSTUFF YOU CAN ALSO USE ON YOUR SKIN

List of beauty products you can also eat

Many culinary oils can be used to make moisturizers for your skin. In the following list of vegetable oils I have marked these with an asterisk (*). (See pages 93-95 for cosmetic uses of vegetable oils.) The following vegetable oils are also called "good fats," or "essential fats," and using them regularly yields fantastically beautifying and healthy results:

Sunflower oil
Hazelnut oil*
Olive oil*
Brazil nut oil
Safflower oil
Pumpkin seed oil
Avocado oil*
Soya bean oil
Walnut oil

Linseed and flaxseed oils have omega–3, –6, and –9

Both of these oils are great for vegetarians and vegans as a replacement for fish oils, and also make a healthier choice for anyone concerned about the current level of pollution in our seas and its drastic effect on aquatic life.

What do the omega oils do exactly?

Omega oils are also known as EFAs, or essential fatty acids—also known as good fats. Omega–3 and –6 are absolutely essential and cannot be produced within our organism. Therefore, they must be provided by your diet. A limited amount of omega–9 can be produced within the body, provided that the other omegas are present.

Omega oils are useful for:

- Facilitating cell growth and division
- Promoting healthy skin (powerful antioxidant)
- Keeping joints supple
- Lowering blood pressure
- Mood balance during PMT and depression
- Intelligence and behavior (The human brain needs a balance of omega oils to promote the growth of the cerebral cortex, which is responsible for reasoning
- Maintaining good vision
- Strengthening the immune system
- Increasing energy levels, helping to build muscle, and assisting with fat loss

Where to find good quality oils?

They are best purchased cold-pressed and unrefined—meaning that they will not have been extracted at high temperature, which would destroy their health properties, nor will they have been damaged by heavy chemical treatments. Cold-pressed and unrefined are the best oils you can buy, as their natural goodness remains unadulterated. Buy them organic if you really want to treat yourself; that way you will also be able to use them to make your moisturizers. Some supermarkets sell them (not always the organic ones), but health food stores are always a sure supplier. Some brand names of oil mixtures available commercially are very costly, which is great if you can afford it. If you can't or you would like to blend your own, you can choose two or three oils from the list given above.

Oils such as linseed and hemp must be stored in the fridge at all times. All natural oils should be stored away from direct sources of heat and light to protect them from going rancid. Linseed and hemp oils are a great source of vitamins (notably vitamin E), minerals, and omegas 3 and 9—and some also provide omega–6. No oils given in the previous list should be used for cooking with heat, or their properties will be lost, *with the exception of olive oil.*

If you had to choose one oil, olive oil would be the best option

Olive oil, extra-virgin and cold-pressed, is a valuable asset to a healthy lifestyle:

- Its composition remains stable at very high temperatures and does not turn carcinogenic *as all other oils do* when heated, making it a safe and healthy alternative for all types of cooking and frying.
- It contributes to a healthy circulatory system by keeping levels of bad cholesterol low, while nourishing the body with essential fatty acids.
- It offers a myriad of health benefits and is *excellent for the skin.*
- Its composition is similar to that of breast milk, making it a wonderful moisturizing oil to heal cracked nipples and totally safe for babies to ingest.

Many cosmetic products are made from olive oil. I once met an elderly lady with such beautiful skin that I felt compelled to ask her what she was using. She said that she could never be bothered with anything complicated and had simply rubbed a little pure olive oil on her face and neck, morning and night, every day of her life. You should have seen the quality of her skin … amazing! It looked and felt (she let me touch it, as she was so proud!) just like a peach.

Tip: The following suggestion will ensure that you take two teaspoons of olive oil on a regular basis. Toast some nice whole meal brown bread, rub a garlic clove over it, and drizzle some oil on top; it makes a nice change from the regular white garlic bread and it is deliciously healthy!

Super-nutritious and beautifying vinaigrette

This recipe will provide an intake of several good fats. You'll need:

One soupspoon of coarse (or any) mustard
One soupspoon of cider or balsamic vinegar (or a little of both)
Two soupspoons each of olive, hemp, and avocado oil
One clove of garlic
Dried herbs (basil, tarragon, or parsley)
Tiny pinch of cayenne or black pepper
One-half teaspoon of soy sauce or pinch of salt (both optional)
One-half teaspoon of honey (optional)

To prepare the vinaigrette:

1. Mix the mustard with the vinegar, and add the soy sauce.
2. Pour in the soupspoons of olive oil very slowly while stirring, then the hemp oil, and finally the avocado oil.
3. Add the grated clove of garlic, the herbs, and the honey. Voila!

You have just made a super-healthy dressing packed with vital nutrients. You can substitute some of the oils with ones you may prefer from the list on page 37. If you are trying to stay away from sugar or honey, it is easy, as the balsamic vinegar has a sweetness of its own. You can leave out the salt, too; it will still be absolutely delicious. If you are using fresh herbs, put them directly on the salad and not in the dressing, as the vinegar "cooks" them and makes them limp.

Store your vinaigrette in a glass and put it in the fridge for use as needed.

A word of caution: Please note that the sunflower oil (and most other oils) you find at your local supermarket is *usually not* cold-pressed and in fact *highly refined*. Be sure to check the bottle and avoid using any such oils, especially if you are prone to high cholesterol and/or trying to lose weight. Never use that kind of oil for massage or to moisturize your body or face.

What about margarine?

There is *absolutely no good reason* to use margarine, *ever*! If you want something that tastes like butter, have butter … or don't. Margarine, and anything else that contains hydrogenated fats, cannot be processed any further by the body, so it clogs up the arteries.

Tip: Some cake recipes lend themselves to swapping the use of margarine for one of the nut oils. Experiment with walnut, hazelnut, or Brazil nut oil in your favorite recipes—it works!

A note of caution regarding the *abstinence from good fats*

Many people who wish to lose weight tend to indiscriminately eliminate all fats from their diet, including "good fats". Sadly, most of those are women wishing to remain slim and beautiful. Such an obsession with banning all fats from their diet is a dangerously negative decision that is sure to lead to serious physical and mental deficiencies and, of course, cost them the very thing they treasure most: *their youthful good looks!*

Abstinence from EFAs will contribute to the following:

- The development of mental illnesses: anything from postpartum depression to Alzheimer's disease.
- Putting on weight—THAT'S RIGHT! The "good fats" (also called good cholesterol) repair damage done by the "bad fats" (also called bad cholesterol) and contribute to their elimination.
- Faulty cardiovascular system, immune system, and nervous system.
- Breakdown of organ function, and ACCELERATED AGING.

So think twice about refusing half an avocado or a spoon of flaxseed oil.

OTHER BEAUTIFYING FOODS, FOR EATING ONLY!

Raw wisdom as a natural prescription for beauty

Eating a good amount of *raw fruits and vegetables* on a daily basis is vital for vibrant health. All vegetables lose a lot of their enzymes and precious vitamins when boiled and become limp and lifeless, which is tasteless and off-putting. It is better to steam them if you want to eat them cooked, with the exception of potatoes of course and a few other root vegetables, which are better fully boiled. You don't need any fancy cooking equipment unless you really want to buy a steamer. Simply put a little water (1 inch) in the bottom of any saucepan and keep the lid on to steam. You will feel an upsurge of energy when you start to include some raw wisdom in your diet.

Eating raw food in winter or in colder climates can be challenging, but a colorful and crispy salad is always seductive! Think of it as your natural prescription to aging gracefully. Why not try some of the following: rocket, spinach, watercress, thinly grated carrots, avocado, thinly grated raw beetroot and celeriac, celery, tomatoes (fresh or sun-dried) cucumber, endives, onions, peppers, asparagus, slivers of mushrooms, etc. The list is endless!

Don't forget to sprinkle some sprouted seeds on your salad.

Tip: If you are not keen on eating too many raw vegetables or have trouble digesting them, you may steam them very quickly: one or two minutes will ensure that most vitamins are still present.

Divine carrot salad

You'll need:

Three organic carrots
One-half lemon
One inch of fresh ginger root
One clove of garlic
Dried raisins or fresh grapes (optional)

To prepare:

1. Simply grate the carrot using the thin side of the cheese grater.
2. Squeeze the lemon juice over the carrots.
3. Grate the garlic clove and the ginger root.
4. Mix all together. That's it!

Note: Keep this in the fridge so that it is fresh and juicy. It is absolutely delicious and full of beautifying goodness, even children love it! If you are using raisins, store the salad in the fridge for a few hours; the moisture from the carrots and the lemon juice will have rehydrated the raisins, which will be plump and juicy. Yum!

NEED A BOOST?

Avocados are a creamy and silky treat that nourish your skin and give it a smooth and velvety quality. They are quite high in fat, but do not worry, as it is the good kind! Avocadoes are rich in potassium and vitamins B, E, and K.

Tip: If your skin feels very dry and lifeless, add half an avocado to your diet *every day* for a whole week. This will dramatically improve the condition of your skin. A little lime or lemon juice poured over the avocado will stop it from oxidizing and complement your intake of vitamin C.

Onions have great healing and cleansing properties, and they are also a great immune-boosting food. Eaten raw or cooked, onions act as an antiseptic; clear the blood of unhealthy fats (bad cholesterol); can counteract fluid retention; and help to prevent heart attacks, break down mucus congestion, and fight against free radicals (for more information on free radicals, see page 23).

Tip: If you are making your own fresh juice at home, add half a small onion to it. Otherwise, thinly chop the same amount and add over your salad or into your vinaigrette.

Garlic also has fantastic cleansing, toning, and healing properties; I am not just saying that because I am French ... honestly! It contains selenium, which helps to boost the immune system and promotes the elimination of free radicals. It can be eaten raw or cooked, although eating it raw would have the most positive impact on your health. It has antiviral, antifungal, and antibacterial properties. A great boosting food for the immune system, it acts as a powerful antioxidant and can help in the prevention of cancer. It cleanses the blood, helps to lower cholesterol, and prevents blockages in the arteries; it is also an antiseptic. Garlic is another powerful ally that helps you to stay beautifully young and in top condition!

Tip: Finely grate a clove of garlic into your salad or vinaigrette for easier absorption. Chew on a coffee bean or some parsley if you don't like the smell it leaves on the breath. If you really can't eat garlic at all, consider getting it as a supplement in the form of odorless capsules.

Ginger is a great digestive aid; it has warming and stimulating qualities (see page 153 for the detoxifying ginger bath). It is also a great decongestant when you have a cough, a cold, or the flu. Ginger clears the mind with its invigorating properties and acts as a great tonic for the reproductive system, for men and women alike. It is even believed to be an aphrodisiac!

Tip: You can make an excellent tea by grating a teaspoon of fresh ginger root into boiling water. Immediately reduce the heat and leave the root to simmer for about ten minutes. The wise women of Africa have enjoyed ginger root tea for centuries; they know about its soothing properties that are so beneficial during difficult menstruation.

Alternatively, you can simply add a little grated ginger root to a warming winter vegetable casserole or a stir-fry. It may spice up more than your dinner!

Cayenne pepper qualifies as a super-antioxidant with its high content of vitamin C and beta-carotene—a real ally when it comes to keeping the free radicals at bay and delaying the effects of aging. It also protects your body-temple against degenerative illnesses such as cancer and from cardiovascular disease. It has a positive effect on the mind, triggering a sense of well-being and slight euphoria due to the endorphins produced on contact with your tongue. Use in moderation, as always.

Tip: Cayenne pepper can be added to any dish you like; just make sure that you only use a tiny amount (about the size of a match's head for one serving) *after* your food is cooked, especially for those of you who have a delicate stomach.

Turmeric is a deliciously warm and sensual spice and a *very powerful* antioxidant. It has anti-inflammatory properties; it helps to protect the liver; and it is very beneficial in the prevention of cancer. You can buy turmeric in capsule form or simply use a little of the powdered spice in your meals. It is widely used in Indian food.

Algae and seaweed might not be in your pantry, but they certainly deserve to be. They are both members of the royal family when it comes to *antioxidants*. They are packed with nutrients and promote cell regeneration and repair. Seaweed is a precious gift from the sea, where all life originated.

Algae as a supplement

Have a look around in your local health food store; any of the following produce would benefit you hugely—you need only pick one of them.

There are a few varieties of algae to choose from:

- Spirulina
- Chlorella
- Wild blue-green algae

They are all considered *super-foods* and are usually taken in capsule or powdered form.

Tip 1: Powdered spirulina can be hard to dissolve, as it is very thin powder; so it tends to stay in clumps, which can be unpleasant to drink. To avoid this, use a jar instead of a glass. Put a heaped teaspoon of spirulina powder into a glass of orange juice (or any other juice you might prefer) and shake until thoroughly mixed. You might also like to use a straw to avoid getting green teeth! It doesn't sound very appealing, but believe me, it is worth it; you will look radiant and have tons of extra energy at your disposal.

Tip 2: If you have a tendency to snack between meals and are looking for some help to change that pattern, simply split your spirulina shake in two dosages and use it as a snack. Spirulina is high in protein, so it will definitely keep hunger at bay until your next meal. Be prepared for a look of disgust when you pull out your jar at the office and drink your green gooey stuff ... it is not for the faint-hearted!

Edible seaweed

There are many different types of seaweed you can buy, they can be found nearly everywhere nowadays, but definitely in Asian supermarkets as well as in all health food stores. You are probably familiar with sushi, made from rice and raw vegetables or raw fish, rolled in a sheet of seaweed.

Other commonly used seaweeds are:

Agar (can be used instead of gelatin)
Arame
Dulse
Hijiki
Irish moss
Kombu
Nori (to make sushi)
Wakame

Most seaweed can be added to soups and stews, or included to a rice dish for an exotic touch.

Tip: If you find the prospect of cooking with seaweed daunting, you can buy ready-made seaweed flake mixes. Simply sprinkle over soups, salads, pasta, or any other dish. The flakes can replace some of the salt you use in your dishes, as it is very salty. Seaweed is another *super-food* packed full of minerals and vitamins, and it tastes great; could you be tempted?

Probiotic culture (lactobacillus acidophilus bifidobacterium) products are great for a balanced intestinal flora. They will help to restore inner health for people suffering all kinds of intestinal discomforts such as constipation, upset stomach, or irritable bowel syndrome (IBS), and they help to replenish the depletion of good bacteria after a course of antibiotics. Constipation is a serious enemy of good health and should be banned altogether. Please go to page 66 for more handy tips on the subject; I devoted a whole section on it because it is such a common issue. A daily dose of yogurt, for example, with live culture (make sure you check the ingredients) will help the intestinal transit time. It would be better to buy something that does not have any sugar in it, especially if you suffer from thrush or any other symptoms related to *Candida albicans*. Fresh fruits can be added to yogurt, and a little honey may be used if you have no health issues, but plain yogurt is also fine. If you are eating something spicy, a little bowl of yogurt will bring down the fire.

Tip: Be aware that most probiotic products available commercially are laced with sugar and may do more harm than good. Natural organic yogurt is cheaper and much more effective.

Kefir is a healthy and therapeutic alternative to yogurt; it is packed full of enzymes that are extremely beneficial for the intestinal flora and has a natural sweetness of its own. It is available in most Eastern European food stores, or you can buy the culture to make it at home.

Produce hosting live culture is widely available today; you can even buy live frozen yogurt, which is very tasty. Some other products such as granola bars, candy bars, cereals, and cookies are said to have live cultures, and maybe they do. Personally, I prefer to have the "real thing" in yogurt, free from excessive, sickly sweetness. The choice is yours.

Tip: Health food stores sell the same live cultures as supplements for those who have a dairy intolerance. If you have been ill and under antibiotic treatment, you may need a huge dose of live cultures, in which case taking it as a supplement may be more practical. Store your acidophilus supplement in the fridge at all times.

Fish and shellfish are brilliant, and think about it: shellfish and some other fish feed on algae and seaweed! Eating some fish or shellfish two or three times a week is a real treat for your heart, your arteries, your brain (handy to retain good memory), your skin, and sometimes your sex drive (oysters are thought to have aphrodisiac properties—if eating them doesn't turn you off first!). One of my favorites is wild Alaskan salmon, which has a much darker flesh due to the quality of the seaweed on which it feeds. Tuna, herring, mackerel, sea bass, trout, etc., are all delicious and extremely good for you. Make sure they are either fresh or just packed in brine, and not in cheap oil, as is often the case with tinned tuna. It is wise to consume a minimum of smoked fish (and any other smoked foods), as it is carcinogenic due to the presence of smoke molecules in the flesh. Again, moderation is a great thing… there is no harm in eating smoked produce on special occasions.

Tip: Sardines are surprisingly good for you, too, and *very affordable* if you are on a budget.

Seafood is generally lower in fat, with the exception of certain species of shrimp. Generally, all seafood contains all the super-beneficial vitamins and minerals and the omega oils you require for optimal health, vitality, and beautiful skin.

Tip: If you are conscious about your weight or simply wish to eat your fish or shellfish without heavy sauces (which are usually made with butter and cream—delicious but deadly!), why not try the following cooking method.

Simple and healthy cooking alternative for fish

1. Put the fish of your choice (or scallops) in a pan with a little olive oil.
2. Squeeze half a lemon or lime over it.
3. Sprinkle with soy sauce (or salt).
4. Grind some pepper and sprinkle to taste.
5. Put a lid on the pan, so the mixture gently steams.

As the dish cooks, a wonderful juice develops. This is a winner for the whole family! Poaching, baking, or the light frying method offered above are all healthier ways to eat fish. Moreover, these methods ensure that the omega oils are still present when you enjoy your meal.

Deep -frying kills most of the precious nutrients in the fish and should be kept to an absolute minimum.

Meat really ought to be bought organic, or free-range at least, even if that means it is eaten less often. In certain countries it is common to eat meat every day, at lunch and dinner. This type of consumption is a fast track to acquiring gout, not good health! If you care for your health at all, eating meat two or three times a week is plenty.

Another important fact to consider is that, if a lot of animal protein is consumed on a regular basis and there is no regular bowel elimination, the meat rots in the gut, providing a breeding ground for *many serious illnesses*. Some meat is not worth eating at all, ever: I am sure that you have come across cheap battery-caged chicken ... absolutely terrible—and the rubbery texture doesn't even come close to real meat. A can of beans or a bowl of brown rice would be safer and tastier than any dish made with mass-produced animal protein.

Tip: Some meat is leaner than others; why not try quail, venison, pheasant, or rabbit? A good organic chicken is absolutely wonderful; treat yourself once in a while. Why not replace one or two of your meat dishes with a fish dish each week?

Brewer's yeast is probably the richest natural source of all B vitamins and folic acid you can find (together with Marmite spread) and is a great food that promotes cell repair and maintains your health and beauty. Brewer's yeast is also a great source of zinc, which is said to be particularly important for the optimal functioning of the male sex organs, and helps to keep the prostate in top condition. Zinc also keeps mental and physical processes at their most efficient. Brewer's yeast contains selenium, which acts as an important *aging-prevention mineral.*

Tip: Simply sprinkle a spoonful over your soup or any other dishes you like. Vegans use it as a replacement for cheese over pizzas, pastas, etc.

Legumes (such as beans, peas, and lentils) are a great source of nutritional antioxidants. They contain the good fats, B vitamins, and plenty of fiber, and they provide long periods of energy due to their slow release into your system.

Here are a few different kinds of beans that are delicious:

Adzuki beans
Butter beans
Black beans
Kidney beans
Garbanzo beans (chickpeas)
Lentils (green, red, brown, or yellow)

Mung beans
Soybeans (tofu, soymilk, and miso are all made from soybeans)

Tip: Are you worried about flatulence? It's not a good enough reason not to eat beans; they are so good for you! Besides, there are a couple of things you can do to make sure that you keep that problem at bay:

- Always soak the legume, whichever one you choose, for a full twelve hours. Change the water once in that period of time if you know that your stomach has difficulties digesting legumes.
- Cook your beans in water thoroughly until soft.

When you use your cooked beans to make the dish of your choice, *add some fresh herbs*. Some of them promote easier digestion, in particular, parsley, dill, fresh coriander, or chives. Herbs all have great healing properties and add a lot of flavor to your meal. You can use them to prepare casseroles, hummus, and soups or serve them cold with a salad. Legumes are another handy addition to your lunchbox while working or traveling.

TOPICS EXPLORED IN SECTION 3

- Vegetable oils you can eat and use to make your moisturizers
- Do you eat "good fats"?
- Make your own beautifying vinaigrette
- Divine carrot salad
- Do you need a boost?
- Does your home-cooked food include a varied menu made of super-nutrients?
- Simple and easy cooking alternative for fish

NOTES

4. To Take or Not To Take Vitamins: That is the Question!

If we lived in an ideal world ...

Where everything was home-grown and certified organic, AND there wasn't so much pollution ... and if, and if! This isn't the case for most of us, so you see where this is going ... we probably wouldn't need any vitamins. However, in the world that we live in, most of us don't eat fully organic foods or have stress-free lives, so it really is up to you if you want to take supplements or not. You might have read many conflicting statements on the subject, which can be very confusing. The people who sell vitamins tell us that we absolutely need them—and so many of them! Some research shows that the body has trouble extracting nutrients that are not in natural form. You may have noticed that when you take some vitamins, urine takes on a strong color and odor.

Personally, I choose to take the *middle road,* as I figure that even if the absorption percentage is far smaller than the intake, it is definitely better than none. I feel that it is best to assist the body by taking certain vitamins to sustain good health and prevent deficiencies, especially after the age of thirty-five. Don't get me wrong, good nutrition is vital and there are absolutely no shortcuts! The result—how healthy and vibrant you feel (and look)—very much depends on how you treat yourself as a whole. *Your most important responsibility* is to take care of yourself; the better you feel the more energy you have at your disposal, especially for those of you who are taking care of young children, sick family, and elders.

Do check with your health practitioner before you self-diagnose and buy your own supplements randomly

Apart from anything else, it will save you buying too much of the same kind. Certain supplements enhance the absorption of others, so be sure you talk to someone who is qualified to answer your questions; the staff at most health food stores is knowledgeable and can be very helpful.

A note of caution

- Those of you who have health problems must definitely consult your GP before taking any supplements.
- Anyone feeling seriously depleted of energy should have a blood test done, rather than relying on self-diagnosis and possibly taking the wrong supplements.
- There is such a thing as toxicity from too much vitamins and, in some cases, it can become a serious health hazard. For example, vitamins that are fat-soluble are processed through the liver and should not be taken excessively—so ask for advice.

Tip: It is well worth spending *good money for good vitamins* extracted from natural sources (available in all good health food stores) as *cheap vitamins give cheap effects*. The golden rule is that vitamins should be taken with food to aid your system in assimilating them.

VITAMINS AND MINERALS FOR A GLOWING BODY-TEMPLE

The vitamins covered here are not, by any means, the only ones that your body may require if you have different health issues. We are mainly exploring the supplements that are helpful in slowing down the aging process and maintaining your health and beauty.

THE VITAMINS

VITAMIN E is considered to be one of the most significant contributors when it comes to *anti-aging nutrients*. Vitamin E is an all-powerful natural antioxidant that helps to keep your skin supple and radiant. We covered a vast amount of food that provides the body with plenty of vitamin E (see pages 37-39), but if you want to top-up your intake, you can also take it as a supplement. It is said to work in the prevention, repair, and regeneration of cell damage, as it inhibits the formation of free radicals in the body.

VITAMIN A is another powerful antioxidant; it works in conjunction with Vitamin E. Vitamin A improves cell oxygenation by helping nutrients to be carried out to every cell in your body: the ultimate secret of youth. It keeps your skin soft, strong, and supple, and free from blemishes.

Caution: Do respect the suggested dosage, as an excessive intake of vitamin A will show up as a strong orange tint on the inside of your hands and feet, and leave you looking like an Oompa-Loompa!

VITAMIN C is a very important vitamin. In fact, if you only wanted to take one vitamin, *this would be a really good one to choose*. It is said to be our most powerful ally when it comes to eliminating toxins. Vitamin C is water-soluble and *is not stored in the body,* so taking it as a supplement is a must. It is paramount in assisting your immune system; *a good daily supply will help to ensure that you are never sick*. Vitamin C is vital for collagen formation, it is a superb antioxidant, and it helps to keep your blood vessels strong and clean. It works in conjunction with vitamin A and E, aiding the body with the assimilation of nutrients. Vitamin C helps with the absorption of iron, so a glass of orange juice is great with a spinach salad or a good helping of parsley. Vitamin C is safe to ingest in relatively large doses; the only side effect of taking too much of it is diarrhea, in which case you can reduce your dosage a little. Vitamin C is very easily destroyed by, for example: smoking, drinking, stress, regular exposure to neon lighting, sunbeds, too much sun, pollution, etc.

Do you smoke and/or drink regularly?

Then do yourself a HUGE favor and take some good quality vitamin C *every day*. You can take it up to three times per day; a total of 4,000 to 6,000 mg (4 to 6 g) is perfectly safe. I am not talking about the fizzy tablets, because if you try taking a high dosage of those, you will be so full of gas that you might take off! Buy ascorbic acid, which is pure vitamin C in powder form.

Tip: Half a spoon of pure vitamin C powder mixed in some orange juice will give you a 2,500-mg or 2.5-g dose. It is wonderfully efficient and costs a fraction of the price of any other form of vitamin C. Don't let anybody tell you otherwise; any vitamin in pill form is loaded with bulking agents, which are mainly used to keep its shape. Vitamin C with bioflavonoid has become very fashionable and consequently very pricey. The bioflavonoids facilitate the absorption and use of vitamin C by the body, which you can replicate yourself at home by mixing your powdered vitamin C with orange juice. It can be taken morning, noon, and evening: a 2000-mg (2-g) dose each time is safe and very effective. It beats the time-released over-priced vitamin!

If you don't drink or smoke, you can still take the same dosage or slightly less if you wish, depending on your lifestyle and diet. You will observe *powerful rejuvenating effects* on your skin, and you will rarely be sick.

A note of caution: Use a straw to drink the vitamin C mixed in juice; it is very acidic and can eventually contribute to damaging the enamel on your teeth.

Interesting fact: Linus Carl Pauling was an American quantum chemist and biochemist (1901–1994) and twice a Nobel Prize winner. He advocated the benefits of taking much larger amounts of vitamin C than are acceptable according to the RDA (recommended daily allowances): over 2,000 mg (20 g) per day. While I am not saying that you should do that, this may reassure you on taking a 400- to 600-mg dose daily. Do a little extra research yourself if you are curious about its many uses.

VITAMIN B-COMPLEX is another treasure you may like to acquire while on your health and beauty quest. It is a cocktail of several B vitamins that are essential for good health; it offers protection from stress, promotes cell growth and division, improves circulation, and can increase sexual stamina and keep reproductive organs healthy. It helps to keep the skin, hair, and nails in top condition, as it protects the cells from oxidation, thus halting the aging process. It also contributes to the optimal functioning of the brain and can have a beneficial role in the prevention of heart problems.

THE MINERALS

SELENIUM is said to be one of the most potent minerals when it comes to antioxidants. It is a powerful contributor to the elimination of free radicals in the body. Selenium is present in garlic and onions, seafood, brewer's yeast, rice, chicken, tuna, eggs, and Brazil nuts (very high), and is also available in health food stores as a supplement. Always check the prescribed dosage so you do not exceed the RDA. Selenium has been found to protect the body from certain forms of cancer, especially breast cancer. It can help the body cleanse itself of toxins, especially mercury poisoning.

ZINC, CALCIUM, AND MAGNESIUM are all extremely important minerals for radiant health. They all contribute to your body's finely tuned system so it keeps working in top condition. These minerals are essential for cell division and cell growth; they assist the natural process of detoxification and keep your bones and teeth strong and healthy. Zinc, calcium, and magnesium can be taken as supplements but are also found in many different types of food such as seeds and nuts, dark leafy vegetables, meat, fish, etc.

TOPICS EXPLORED IN SECTION 4

- Check your diet: do you need to use vitamins and minerals?
- Do you smoke and drink regularly?

NOTES

5. Herbs and Teas

Mother Nature has blessed us with an abundance of amazing herbs

Herbs have been used since prehistoric times and were once the only form of medicine available. Because they work extremely well and are very potent, it is best to look for a qualified herbalist practitioner if you want to get real results. They will give you a tailor-made herbal mix to suit your individual needs, and you will find the benefits astonishing. Some herbs can also be purchased directly from health food stores, either loose—so, for example, you can make your own herbal teas—or as supplements. All options are good. As always, choose the best quality you can find, organic or wild-grown are superior, as they haven't been treated with pesticides.

Tip: If you have no health problems and simply want to take a tonic for *a boost in the spring or the autumn*, a good cocktail of herbs can really do wonders for the mind, the body, and the spirit! Find a reputable herbalist and give yourself the gift of health. This is also great as a tonic for teenagers who have to cope with their developing bodies and are probably going through stressful times during studies and exams.

A SUPER-POWERFUL HERBAL EXTRACT

GRAPE SEED EXTRACT/ PINE BARK EXTRACT (Pycnogenol) Research shows that its antioxidant properties are fifty times greater than those of vitamins E and C, making it a brilliant asset when it comes to *anti-aging* herbal supplements. Grape seed extract can also contribute to wound healing; it can help to lower bad cholesterol and prevent varicose veins; and it plays a role in improving eyesight, protects the heart, and enhances brain function. In men, it can contribute toward sexual health and performance, and is also helpful for maintaining an erection and increasing sperm count. For women, it is beneficial for difficult menstruation and it can assist with the healing of post-gynecological surgery. This is an herb and not a vitamin, so you can take it while using other supplements. No known contra-indications have been found, to date.

MORE WONDERFUL HERBS

MILK THISTLE protects and repairs the liver, which is essential if you regularly consume alcohol and/or experience regular bouts of anger. It can be taken as part of a maintenance program for a period of two or three weeks once or twice a year.

BILBERRY is another powerful antioxidant. It promotes good blood circulation, and improves and prevents problems related to the eyes.

GINKGO BILOBA is a great antioxidant. It is said to aid blood circulation to organs and tissue, and to help maintain optimal memory function. *Do not take before surgery,* as it can thin out the blood.

WHAT ABOUT BLACK, GREEN, AND WHITE TEAS?

They can certainly contribute to your health. It should be noted, however, that they are all diuretics and should be used sparingly. These teas certainly cannot replace the amount of water the body needs and therefore do not count toward the six to eight glasses recommended on a daily basis. In fact, you should drink an extra glass of water with each cup of tea or coffee to avoid dehydration. The following analyses are based on a serving of eight ounces of water over the tea bag of your choice:

Black Tea has an average of 40 mg of caffeine per serving.

Green Tea has an average of 20-plus mg of caffeine per serving.

White Tea has an average of 15 mg of caffeine per serving.

The black, green, and white teas have indisputable *antioxidant properties*. Green and white teas are particularly well known for their detoxifying qualities. White tea has been found to have two to five times more antioxidants than green tea. White tea is the least processed of all the teas and can be more palatable than the green variety, as it is lighter. All the above teas are best consumed without milk.

Tip: To obtain maximum benefit from the green and white teas you drink, the hot water used to make the beverage should be allowed to cool down to just below the boiling point. This prevents the hard and bitter taste that green tea can develop while brewing.

As with everything else that becomes popular, it can be thought that the more of it you drink, the healthier you become. Not so. Too much, even of a good thing, is still too much! One or two cups of green or white tea a day can be an asset for your health; any more tea will simply dehydrate your body.

HERBAL TEAS, such as chamomile, sage, peppermint, yarrow, nettle, lemon, verbena, etc., contain no caffeine at all. They are very tasty and also have individual healing properties. See pages 149-150 for detoxifying properties of herbs.

COFFEE has an average of 80-plus mg of caffeine per serving.

Tip: A pinch of cinnamon mixed in a cup of black coffee helps to burn fat. The bitter quality of this beverage acts as a tonic for the liver.

TOPICS EXPLORED IN SECTION 5

- How much regular tea and coffee do you drink?
- The use of herbal supplements as antioxidants
- A look at black, green, and white tea

NOTES

6. Constipation: Enemy of Good Health and Glowing Skin

How do you know if you are constipated?

Aside of the obvious lack of bowel movement for any amount of time (starting with one day), the *quality* of your bowel movement is very important. Before so much medical technology was available, doctors used to enquire about the patient's bowel habit, color, and frequency, as this alone can reveal much about one's health. Some doctors still do, but most, unfortunately, do not. You can take care of your own health by paying close attention to this yourself or by consulting a natural practitioner if the advice offered here isn't sufficient for you.

If the bowel content is retained in the body, the toxins that haven't been eliminated are reabsorbed and carried back to the liver, which can cause many health problems ranging from benign to very serious.

Check list:

- You should have one or more bowel movement *every day.* Depending on the frequency and the amount of food eaten each day, one or two bowel movements are normal and, in fact, necessary.
- The quality of the bowel movement is also very important. Stools should be soft enough and be in the shape of an *S*, which is the shape of the end of your colon.
- Floating stools are not indicative of good fiber intake and could, in fact, signify poor absorption of the nutrients ingested.
- Any bowel movement that is "knotted" (like sheep's stools), dry, and painful to pass is indicative of constipation, *even if it occurs regularly.*

Tip: If you are eating relatively well most days but still find yourself constipated, it might be worth keeping a diary of the food you eat. This way, you can begin to identify what food is responsible for clogging up your system. This is a simple and effective way to understand your own body mechanism so you can make the necessary changes to start living a more comfortable life. The emotional side of constipation may be that you are holding onto to something or someone; so look within to see if there are influences from which you need to free yourself. It may be old beliefs; check within to feel what is holding up the flow in your life. Becoming aware of any unwanted influences will assist the letting-go process in itself. See the emotional cleanse on page 159 to help you shift unwanted burden. Don't forget to drink plenty of water!

The damage caused by constipation

There is much damage that can be caused by constipation, ranging from benign to very serious. The severity of the damage depends on whether the problem is longstanding and/or chronic.

Here are some issues that may be the result of constipation:

- The skin becomes depleted and lacks luster as it struggles to get rid of toxic overload.
- Feelings of tiredness and irritability
- Terrible bloating
- Backaches
- Headaches
- Depression
- Bad breath and overly strong body odor
- Hemorrhoids
- Varicose veins
- Diverticulitis (buildup of waste logged in pockets of the intestinal wall)
- Colon and prostate cancer

EASY AND PRACTICAL TIPS TO RELIEVE CONSTIPATION

Food and water intake

Extra water, and fiber in the form of fruits, vegetables, and extra whole grains, should be consumed *every day*. Yogurt with live cultures will help too. Refined produce such as white bread, white rice, crackers, etc… *need to be cut out altogether* if you are serious about obtaining healthy and regular bowel habits.

The opposite of constipation is diarrhea, which is just as serious and should be discussed with a health professional, especially if it is a chronic problem. In this case, the body doesn't have time to absorb the vital nutrients ingested, which can result in vitamin deficiency.

HERBS FOR COLON CLEANSING

The following herbs are very useful and completely natural. They make a great alternative to commercial laxatives, as they do not suppress the colon's ability to eliminate regularly and naturally. As a result, these herbs work very effectively, without making the colon lazy or reliant.

The following herbs are in order of strength, starting with the mildest:

Slippery elm: Sold as capsules or powder to make a thick tea.

Cascara sagrada: Available in capsules and liquid herb extract.

Senna pods: Start with five or six pods to begin with; brew in boiling hot water and drink as tea. If you find that this does not have the required effect, add a few more pods—but take it easy, it really is very strong!

Tip: The good news is that they all work very well; so don't plan on a shopping spree for about five to seven hours after taking a tea made from these herbs. The best thing is to have it the night before, or in the morning if you can stay at home for the next few hours. The result and amount of time needed for a successful colon cleanse very much depends on your organism and the severity of your constipation.

SEEDS FOR COLON CLEANSING

The effect of these seeds is slightly gentler in cleansing action; however, it would be wise to try them out while at home. This way, you can see how your system reacts.

Ground Flaxseeds can be added to soups, yogurt, or cereals. Just bear in mind that it absorbs water very fast, turning into a kind of jelly, so anything you mix it in will bulk up and bind. This is how it works inside the colon: the cleansing bulk assists in taking the waste down.

Psyllium seeds can also be left overnight to bulk up in water and can be added to juice or soup, or simply taken by teaspoon and chased down with a large glass of water.

Psyllium husks are equally efficient and are available in capsule form. Alternatively, a teaspoon full of husks can be added to a glass of fruit juice or a smoothie.

Exercises to help the elimination of constipation

COLON MASSAGE

This exercise is practiced in bed, as it is more effective when done while lying down. Start by applying quite deep pressure in a clockwise motion, starting from the bottom right side of your abdomen (just inside your hip bone) and working your way all around the colon, finishing at the bottom of your left side. Pay special attention to the corners of the colon under the ribs, where the waste is often held up, causing blockages. Repeat several times, morning and night, for *guaranteed results*. With a little experience, you will be able to feel where the blockages are in the colon and apply more localized pressure, ensuring immediate elimination.

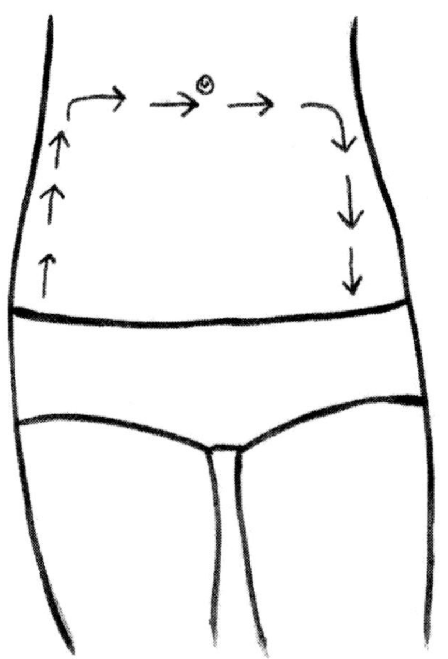

COLON ACUPRESSURE POINTS

There are a series of acupressure points that you can use to stimulate your bowels. They are found between the navel and the pubic bone. Simply start by applying firm pressure with both thumbs, each of them one inch away from your belly button. Stay on each pressure point for one or two minutes and work your way down until you reach your pubic bone as illustrated bellow.

Tip: With both of these exercises, you may feel your bowels moving almost immediately. To ensure prompt and regular success, drink a glass of water on rising; it will help you to eliminate on a daily basis, one or more times. You'll feel lighter than ever, with renewed energy, a kick in your step, a sparkle in your eyes, and glowing skin!

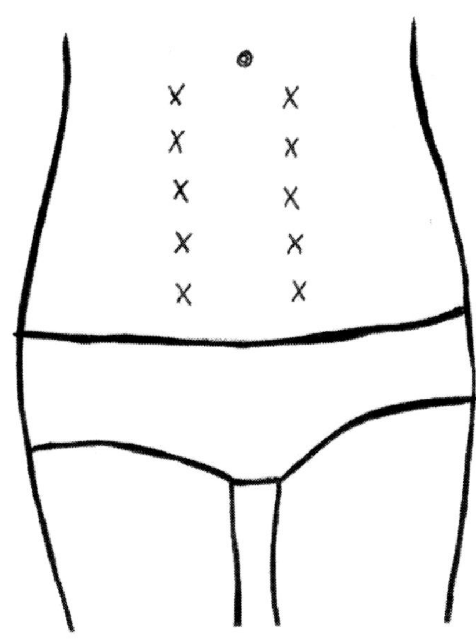

TOPICS EXPLORED IN SECTION 6

- Do you suffer from constipation?
- Symptoms and ill effects of constipation
- Herbs and other tips to remedy constipation
- Exercises to eliminate constipation

NOTES

7. The Gift of Sleep

A good night's sleep is one of the simplest and most effective rejuvenating secrets

Readily available anytime, you can decide on the quality and the duration of the rest you give yourself. This section can also fit in the "Free Rejuvenating Secrets" chapter, as there is no extra charge for a nap or a good night's sleep: the best things in life are free! While you are asleep, your conscious mind is not in the way, which means that natural divine intelligence can do its job, and much-needed regeneration takes place.

HOW MUCH SLEEP DO YOU NEED?

This very much depends on the individual. It varies according to personality type—some of us are "night-people" and are more alive in the evening and others are morning people, brighter early on in the day. The kind of work you do, how much sports or other vigorous activity you perform each day, the food you consume before bedtime, the amount of stress you experience, etc., all play a part in how much rest you really need; there is no set rule. People who practice regular meditation find that they need less sleep, as the body is regenerated through relaxation, and stress is kept to a minimum. One thing is for sure: we all need a certain amount of regular sleep to function with good grounding and to look and feel refreshed!

Sleeping posture

If you don't feel refreshed enough upon awakening, check the following few points to see if you can help yourself. Try sleeping on your back with a good pillow:

- The back gets a chance to realign itself (see page 130-132 on the Alexander Technique for more information regarding your back).

- Puffiness around the eyes can be reduced, as there is no obstruction to lymph drainage around the neck and face.
- The skin on the face can smooth itself out overnight if not crunched into pillows (which also absorbs all your moisturizer!).

"Bags" under the eyes are very unappealing, mainly for the person wearing them, and no miracle cream can replace those precious hours of much-needed rest. It is said that each hour of sleep before midnight is worth two or three after that; and I must say that I have experienced that to be true. An average of six to eight hours of sleep is what most of us need to recharge our batteries. Give your body a good chance to replenish itself; it is at your disposal all day, so it deserves a comfortable break!

WHAT ABOUT HEATING IN THE BEDROOM?

If you want to feel well rested and look refreshed, don't use any heating in the bedroom!

Heating overnight depletes your whole system, dries your skin and your throat, and leaves you with a groggy feeling upon awakening. You wake up feeling (and sometimes looking) like you've swallowed a whole cactus sitting in the Sahara Desert. Hotel rooms can be terribly stuffy in the winter. Even if you are in a really cold climate, you are far better off using extra blankets and a hot water bottle to help you generate your own body heat.

Tip: If there is no way you can turn off the heat and you can't bring yourself to keep the windows open for fear of wasting precious resources or contributing to global warming (and you would be right), simply put a wet towel over the radiator. This will provide some amount of moisture in the air and keep you reasonably hydrated while you sleep.

WHAT ABOUT PILLOWS?

If you wake up to swollen, puffy eyes

You might benefit from investing in a really good pillow. There are all sorts to choose from, just like mattresses: orthopedic, memory foam, feather down, etc. The main thing is that you find a pillow that is a good fits for you and supports your head properly. There are plenty of conflicting reports and opinions on the subject among back-care specialists, so let us use common sense and personal preference. Simply observe that when you are in an upright position and standing against a wall in a natural manner (not forcedly straight like a pole), there is some space between the back of your head and the wall, whereas your back is making full contact with the wall. That space is indicative of the required thickness of the pillow you need to support your head properly for maximum comfort: not too high and not too low. If your main sleeping position consists of resting on your side, then the same principle applies and is, in fact, even more important. Otherwise the body is "crushed" on itself, the spine gets distorted, and you feel aches and pains in the neck and shoulders upon awakening.

Having no pillow at all—although some prefer this way of sleeping—can cause blockages around the top vertebrae, constricting breathing and reducing the natural blood flow and lymphatic drainage to the head, which can result in increased snoring, exhaustion, back pain, or puffy eyes.

Tip: Find the right pillow *for you*.

- If you sleep on your side, find a pillow that fills the gap and supports you comfortably between the side of your head and your shoulder.
- If you sleep on your back, finding the right pillow means that your chin should not be on your chest, and your head should not be tilted back. Your head must be in alignment with your spine.

You might get strange looks in the store while you are seeking and trying the perfect pillow … but this is nothing compared to an uncomfortable night's sleep and a stiff neck! Just keep smiling at the sales assistant.

UNABLE TO GET TO SLEEP?

What you do in the last forty-five minutes before you fall asleep has a huge impact on your mind

So if you have problems getting to sleep, examine what takes place before you retire. It might be a good idea to consider an activity that lends itself to a good night's sleep—or else to use that time to take in information that you need to absorb. Research shows that the last forty five minutes before you fall asleep leave a lasting impression in the subconscious mind overnight, so you can choose to put this time to good use:

- Reading can be great, although it depends on the book's content. Consider swapping suspense stories for easy reading or *cliterature* if you are in the mood!
- A meditation done while lying down is really great to get to sleep.
- Reading over a speech or presentation you have prepared, as it will be absorbed more easily at this time.
- Visualizing your dreams and goals without self limitations.
- Taking a hot bath.
- Enjoying a great lovemaking session!

Get off the "merry go round"

Stress is often the cause of sleeplessness and is a very real threat to good health. The best and quickest way to eliminate it is to enter the present moment. Entering the present moment, or becoming aware, is like finding the button *to switch off* the incoming stress, or having a mini-holiday. (See The "is-ness" exercise on page 143 to help you reconnect to your own peace of mind). Realize that your whole life is made up of continual *present moments;* whatever happens, and whenever it does, it is *always now,* whether you notice it or not.

For example, torturing yourself with what you will tell a coworker or your bank manager tomorrow (which, in reality, never comes) is unnecessary—especially when done at 3:00 a.m., from your bed. Save it for when you meet the person: you can be sure that the speech you have been rehearsing in bed is not what will come out of your mouth by the time you meet him or her. Instead, trust that you will know what to say or do when the moment comes: *right action always comes out of conscious awareness.* For now, enjoy your present situation and location, which is your comfortable bed in your safe bedroom.

Notice your breathing rhythm.

Don't try to alter it; simply notice how shallow it becomes while your head is racing around with stressful thoughts. As you keep paying attention to your breathing, after a short while you will notice that it has become deeper as you become more relaxed, and before you know it, you fall asleep … or at least feel a good deal more relaxed.

Tips: If you notice a pattern of lack of sleep, check what you eat and/or drink before retiring.

- Anything stimulating like tea or coffee should be consumed much earlier in the day: no later than mid-morning, especially if you experience problems falling and staying asleep.
- Make sure two or three hours have elapsed since your last meal.
- Avoid drinking *any water* after 6:00 p.m. if you need to use the bathroom overnight and cannot get back to sleep afterward.

Your body should basically be allowed to wind down to prepare itself to retire.

A simple relaxation to boost your energy level

If you feel your energy levels dipping throughout the day, here is a simple relaxation exercise for you. It is a mixture between a yoga exercise and the traditional "siesta" we take in France after we eat lunch.

- Lie down wherever you can; put a blanket over yourself if you think you are going to get cold.
- Let all thoughts pass you by without judging or analyzing them: don't entertain any of them. See them pass before your witnessing mind, just like the trailers before a movie.
- Let yourself relax for about ten to twenty minutes; half an hour would be better still if it is possible.

You might fall asleep, which is absolutely fine. You can "program yourself" to wake up or become alert again after the time for relaxation is over; you'll be pleasantly surprised at how self-reliant you can be. If, on the other hand, you know that you are going to have a snoring fit because you are exhausted, set an alarm. Those few minutes of rest will give you a welcome boost and keep you going for the rest of the day.

TOPICS EXPLORED IN SECTION 8

- How much sleep do you get?
- What is the quality of your sleep?
- Tips to get a good night's sleep
- Simple relaxation to boost your energy levels throughout the day

NOTES

8. Skin Care: Secrets, Tips and Recipes

Beautifully fresh skin is the greatest beauty challenge of all times

Especially today when everybody wants to look younger and healthier than ever! Whatever is true of any other features, the skin on your face is what shows up first. A clear complexion can be a challenge for some people—if this applies to you because you suffer from regular skin eruptions, your body is probably trying to tell you something important. Problematic skin could be due to hormonal fluctuations (menstruation, PMT, menopause) or stress, but it could also be a reaction to certain foods or drinks, cosmetic products, shaving products, shampoos, etc. You might need to see a qualified natural practitioner or a dermatologist, or you might simply need to change something in your lifestyle. A good kinesiologist, for example, can trace the root of the problem, bypassing your conscious mind and getting accurate information via muscle testing. Look for a list of practitioners in your area.

The skin is our largest excretory system

—Not the bowels, as is commonly believed; please look back at the section on constipation (page 66)for more details on this. If your skin breaks out into spots regularly, it could mean that a lot of toxins are present in your system and are trying to exit the body. Drinking a sufficient amount of water can help your body rid itself of toxic overload. The best thing you can do of course is to make sure you eat and drink what is best for you *most of the time;* we looked at drinks and nutrition extensively on pages 1-65. Consider the following:

- A detox might be in order if you feel the need for a "spring clean" from the inside out; it will certainly restore glowing skin and give you a phenomenal energy boost on completion (see page 147 for detoxifying methods).

- The topical answer to glowing skin is to use a good moisturizer, not omitting to pay special attention to your neck, *as it tends to be forgotten*; there are many cosmetic procedures available for nearly all body parts, but there are actually very few things that can be done for the neck and hands. So don't forget to moisturize several times a day if you need to; prevention is easier, safer, and cheaper!

Tip: Have a hand cream in your bag as hands tend to get washed more than anything else throughout the day. You might also like to have a small tube of eye cream, as this delicate area tends to dry out faster throughout the day.

EXPENSIVE ANTI-WRINKLE CREAMS

We all love them, but does our skin really benefit from them?

I agree that they are a lovely treat to have on the dresser or in the bathroom, and I love having them when I can afford to. The unspoken message they emanate is "I take good care of my skin because I spend huge amounts of money" and "I know how to pamper myself"; or "I simply love to splash out." They make us feel special. The truth is that, while many of them certainly do a very good job at moisturizing the skin, plenty of trials and research have been done proving that they do little more than that. They do not bestow the magical effects they claim to have, so consider:

- If you have plenty of money and want to keep buying them, it's fine, so long as you understand they may not deliver on their promises.
- If you have limited funds, be at peace and know that your skin wouldn't be any better off than if you could afford the most outrageously expensive creams available on the market!

In either case, do yourself a favor and use something really natural *at least half of the time*. The skin can be put under tremendous stress if too many chemicals are used on it. Give it a natural break! See the moisturizers listed on pages 101-102 for wholesome and nourishing recipes I am sharing with you; I have been making my own creams for the past twenty years and am very content with the results.

Tip: You may have come across a skin-care research report that was executed to find the very best and most rejuvenating body moisturizer available on the market today: the result was the beautifully affordable Nivea! That's right: the simple, affordable and traditional body lotion in the blue bottle. So rejoice, those of you on slim budgets: you too can maintain the skin of your dreams! (Just in case you are wondering, I didn't get any sponsorship to convey this information!) Just remember to use your moisturizer daily. Dove is also fantastic, and I love their "Campaign for Real Beauty" ads with all those gorgeous and diverse body shapes. Let us also celebrate the rare occurrence of *integrity* in advertisement!

PREVENTION AND REPAIR

Both are possible, although prevention is always a wiser choice

Do not despair if you have already done a lot of damage to your skin: something can be done for you. Besides all the tips already discussed until now, there are simple steps that can be taken in order to prevent further damage and help restore your natural beauty.

A lot of people focus on cosmetic creams alone, but I have to tell you that this will not be enough if you expect good results *in the long run*. You are made of exquisitely intricate energies, so you would benefit from treating yourself accordingly and not focusing on your physical appearance alone. Your physical appearance will eventually fade, no matter what you do; it is part and parcel of being human; this is why this book talks of inner radiance throughout.

BEAUTY THIEVES

There isn't a single cosmetic cream on the market that can erase what smoking does to your skin

Apart from the obvious life-threatening damage that heavy smoking does to the body (I won't say anything here because you've heard it all before), there are no creams that can get rid of the *grayish and papery* dry look that undoubtedly comes with an overload of toxins in the body. Using a really good moisturizer and having tons of facials and cosmetic treatments may give the skin a momentary luster, but this wears off soon enough, revealing a seriously depleted and prematurely aged complexion. On top of that, new problems can suddenly develop: an excess of oil secretion in some areas (the T-shaped greasy area) this others becoming so dry they take on a leathery quality.

On the other hand, using a very basic and efficient moisturizing cream will have plenty of beneficial effects *if* it is accompanied by a healthy lifestyle including good food, adequate fluid intake, fewer excesses, some exercise, some relaxation time, and a good positive attitude. That is the kind of radiance that simply cannot be bottled. If you really want to look radiant, you have to exercise some amount of self-control and make different choices.

WHAT ARE "AGE" OR "LIVER" SPOTS?

They appear years after over-exposure to sunshine and are not caused by aging nor are they related to liver complaints, as commonly believed

Liver spots are those flat, brown areas that can be found on the face, hands, top of the back, chest, and head (if bald); basically, all the areas that are most exposed to sunlight. While they are not particularly attractive, they are harmless.

A note of caution: Please note that a dark flat area with irregular borders should be checked by your doctor to avert the possibility of melanoma (skin cancer). Liver spots have well defined borders.

Golden secret: Remedy for photo-damaged skin

Here is a little magic that can be used if the damage is already done—assuming, of course, that *adequate care will be taken from now on.* It isn't for everybody, as this product can be a skin irritant and should therefore be used with caution; it is usually prescribed to people who have acne. It cannot be bought over the counter; you need a prescription from your doctor or your dermatologist to get it.

Retin A is a prescription cream which contains retinoid. It is widely used in many cosmetic products, although usually in a much lighter concentration. Have a look next time you check out an anti-aging cream. Retinoids help by unclogging pores, which is why it is also used in the treatment of acne. It basically stimulates the deeper layers of the dermis, causing it to produce renewed skin. It tightens the skin the moment it is applied, and it is also very efficient in considerably reducing the appearance of *age spots,* tightening dilated pores, and smoothing wrinkles that are not too deep. It really *works,* unlike many other cosmetic products sold on the market, full of empty promises. It can be used on the face, the hands, the neck, and the chest. If you want to get rid of a few liver spots in a concentrated area, you can apply it locally several times a week. *Please discuss this with your doctor or dermatologist before using.*

As a rejuvenating treatment, Retin A can be used once or twice a week from your mid-thirties on. Do a small sample application on the inside of your wrist to see if you are able to use it without adverse reactions. Start by using it once per week (or even fortnightly) to see how you react to it, especially if you have very sensitive skin.

Tip: If you find that the Retin A is too strong on its own, mix a little in your night cream (I recommend the "Fountain of Youth" moisturizer on page 100). Some people find that regular anti-wrinkle creams sometimes cause a reaction on their skin, so this method ensures that you use the exact amount your skin can take.

Warning, to be respected without exception

The use of sunscreen is *absolutely necessary* when using Retin A cream. The skin will be prone to increased photo-sensitivity while it is working on renewing itself. The best thing to do is to use it overnight. In the morning, use rose water as your cleanser/toner on a cotton wool pad for best results and apply your moisturizer before your SPF (Sun Protection Factor) cream. Use your foundation last. If you are using a foundation that has an SPF in it, do please still use a good-quality SPF cream under it, as that in a foundation is never strong enough to protect your skin.

BASIC AND OPTIMAL SKIN REGIME FOR MEN AND WOMEN

Do you want to have radiant skin, supple and soft?

You won't believe how simple the whole affair really is; it consists of three easy steps:

1. **PROTECT**
2. **MOISTURIZE**
3. **CLEANSE**

That's it! So let us explore each of these in detail.

1. PROTECT YOUR SKIN

Protecting your skin is one of the most important things you can do, especially because of the environmental issues prevalent today

Using adequate sun protection all year round is very important, the skin specialists tell us, wherever you live and whatever season it is, without exception. However, a more balanced approach to sun exposure may be wise. A certain amount of sunlight is required by your body so that it can produce vitamin D, which is essential for good health. There is no harm in taking a few minutes of sunshine; choose the milder sunrays that shine around sunset or sunrise; fifteen to twenty minutes at the right time of the day is very beneficial.

Is sun protection really necessary?

Sun-induced aging, also known as photo-aging, is the result of too much sun exposure on the skin. The production of precious collagen, which naturally starts to slow down in our thirties, is hindered further by too much sun exposure and can contribute to the skin becoming dull, wrinkled, saggy, and blotchy. Elastin works in conjunction with collagen and provides the skin with its natural elasticity. This is also destroyed with over-exposure to the sun. *And once it's gone … it's gone for good!*

The sun is stronger than ever, due to the damage of the protective atmospheric layers of our beloved planet

A decent sunscreen needs to be applied every day, and in fact several times a day, to protect your skin from harmful sunrays. The factor indication on the packaging tells us how long we stay protected: *it does not last all day*! For example, a sunscreen with an SPF 30 means that you are protected for 30 minutes. Sunscreen products are constantly being refined, and some of them last longer than others; make sure that you use something that is adequate for you. I remember seeing a school teacher featured on a TV show who worked in the same classroom for thirty years, standing in exactly the same spot every day while teaching. Only half of her face had been exposed to sun all that time, and although she had been behind the windows, the side of her face that was exposed to the sun looked considerably weathered—that one side of her face made her look a good ten to fifteen years older than her actual years.

Like a lot of us, I have a habit of leaving my right hand hanging out of the window as I drive. I can only do this for a short two or three months in the summer because I live in Ireland, and there is more rain than sunshine here! My right hand has a considerable amount of *liver spots* compared to my left hand, which is always inside the car. It can be hard to keep applying sun lotion to the hands, as they are frequently washed throughout the day, so this may be another useful thing to keep in your bag. No wonder we girls have the reputation of carrying bags big enough to move house; a girl's got to do what a girl's got to do! Alternatively, or if you are a man, keep a tube in the car.

Don't be fooled by an overcast day: use protection anyway

A lot of cosmetic products contain an SPF 15, which is not always strong enough, especially in foundation. Experts in the field recommend an SPF 30 for everyday use. If you were born with beautiful black skin, then you are blessed with an SPF tremendously higher than those of us with lighter skin. However, if you experience pigmentary changes and are concerned about the health of your skin, use an SPF daily (and have a check up with your doctor immediately).

If you are planning to be exposed to very strong sunlight, a higher protection like an SPF 50 should be used, complete with sun-hat and sunglasses. The damage is usually done many years before it can be seen (which is a shame); otherwise we might have been more careful earlier on.

Tip: If you prefer to use natural products only, there is a wide range of SPFs available on the market today. Choose a sunscreen that has both UVA and UVB for complete protection. UVB rays are the major contributors to sunburns, reddening of the skin and cause damage to the superficial layers of the skin. However they do not penetrate glass, unlike the UVA rays. UVA and UVB rays play an equally key role in the development of skin cancer, and both contribute to tanning and photo-aging. Some creams available in health food stores and some beauty salons have no titanium and zinc oxide, which means that you can avoid the "white shield look" on the protected skin.

Note: Don't forget to protect your children too; their tender skin really needs your attention.

2. MOISTURIZE YOUR SKIN

A good moisturizer needs to be used every day and every night

Equally important, a *very nourishing* cream or oil should be used around the eyes, where the skin is thinner and tends to dry out faster, especially at night. You may use any creams available on the market if you don't want to make your own oil (as offered later in this section); remember that you don't have to spend huge amounts of money to get a good moisturizer—an average of ten to thirty dollars can get you a perfectly good cream.

Tip: Just see how long your skin stays supple throughout the day to determine if what you are using is enough for your skin type. Stay away from any perfumed products, as these often dehydrate delicate skin.

Making your own moisturizer

There is something deeply satisfying about making your own anti-wrinkle cream, especially when it is easy and hassle-free. Remember that you can use some of the oils from your kitchen, as discussed on page 37. Here are some of the added benefits:

- You can change some of the ingredients as your skin improves, so it is stimulated to stay in the best possible condition.
- Your skin benefits from a HUGE BREAK, as it is completely natural.
- They make loving, caring, and handy gifts for your loved ones (aftershave cream, teenager's anti-spot creams, etc.).

There are some simple recipes here, and all relevant information is provided. Making your own moisturizer is like making your own homemade food: it's always better than the commercial stuff. You will feel good about making it, and when you start to use it, you will realize that it is as good as (if not better than) many leading brands of expensive anti-wrinkle creams, and much cheaper!

3. CLEANSE YOUR SKIN

Cleansing your skin couldn't be simpler!

There are hundreds of cleansers and toners available on the market. Many of them are too harsh; some of them do not achieve the promised results. Here is a really simple and easy toner you can make in two quick steps, suitable for all skin types. Both of the base products you need are available from a pharmacy:

- A large bottle of rose water (500 ml)
- A small bottle of witch hazel (125 ml)

Remove a quarter of the rose water from its bottle and replace with witch hazel, enough from the rose water bottle to add between a quarter and a third of witch hazel, three to one ratio.

Save the leftover rose water for making refills. If you are sensitive to witch hazel, simply use much less or leave it out all together. You may use a beautiful colored glass bottle to hold your mix. The rose water is soothing, cleansing, and gently toning; the witch hazel tightens up open pores and clears up congested skin. It provides everything you would expect from a good cleanser and toner.

Do not be put off by such simplicity; it works wonderfully!

Exfoliate once or twice a week to keep your skin at its best

This is for men and women alike—although, admittedly, men exfoliate when they shave; in this case simply exfoliate the parts of your skin that are not shaved. Millions of new cells are produced every second and this leaves quite an accumulation of "dead skin"' waiting to be removed. Although we shed a certain amount naturally, glowing skin is always waiting to be revealed by a good scrub. There are many exfoliating products on the market. *Please note that if you are already using Retin A cream, exfoliating once a week or a fortnight is plenty.* A simple and gentle product should be used. Again, the more expensive products don't seem to do anything extra. Choose a natural scrubbing gel or cream that appeals to you, and leave it someplace where you can see it so that you remember to use it a couple of times per week. It's good to see that exfoliating products are designed and made especially for you too, gentlemen, because we ladies love a soft and cleansed body and face too!

Tip: The best time to exfoliate is under a hot shower. Let the pores of your skin dilate a little for a few minutes under the hot water before you use your scrubbing cream; this allows deeper cleansing. Splash your body and your face with cold water after exfoliating—this tightens the pores and keeps new impurities from settling in straight away.

Homemade exfoliating products

If you are in the mood and have time to make your own scrubbing cream, here are three very quick and easy ways to do just that, using ingredients found in your pantry. And they *really work too*!

* **Mix milk and brown sugar** together and apply to the skin as a scrub. The lactic acid in the milk works as a mild exfoliant, while the sugar scrubs off the dead skin cells. It's easy and effective.

***A mixture of brown sugar and olive oil** can be use to exfoliate your skin naturally. Just put a little oil in your hand and add a teaspoon of sugar. Rub gently on your skin for a few seconds, especially around the nose, the chin, and the forehead. Rinse off with some warm water and feel how beautifully supple and cleansed your skin is!

* **Fresh papaya** performs natural *and gentle* skin abrasion. The papain enzyme found in this delicious fruit literally "eats away" dead skin cells. Many cosmetic manufacturers are aware of this and use papain enzyme in commercial skin peels. At home, simply mash a little papaya and apply directly onto your face; eat the rest, as it is a brilliant antioxidant! Leave on the skin until it dries off, or about twenty minutes, and rinse off with warm water to reveal a glowing, renewed complexion.

BASIC KNOWLEDGE ON CARRIER OILS AND BASE CREAMS

Let's explore a few vegetable oils that you can use to make your own wholesome moisturizer. There will obviously be a few things you need to buy, but then you'll have them on hand when you need to make yourself a refill (and perhaps some vinaigrette as well!).

Base cream

First of all, you need a basic cream to work from. If you are into making your own base cream, this is wonderful, but I will work from a readymade base here, for the sake of time and convenience. If a cream takes too long to make, you won't want to do it.

The following are all good base creams to choose from:

- Aqueous cream
- E 45
- Vegetarian/vegan base (for extra-sensitive skin)

All the moisturizer recipes in this book are made with aqueous cream but these may be substituted with the other two options above or any other good base cream you come across. They are also known as "carrier creams." Aqueous cream and E 45 can be purchased at a pharmacy. The 500-g tub works out to be cheaper and keeps you going while you are experimenting with making your own cosmetic products. Vegetarian and vegan base creams are a little more expensive; they can be purchased from health food stores or aromatherapy clinics. Whatever you choose, use something that is as plain and basic as possible because you are going to add your own ingredients. Synthetic perfumes and additives decrease or negate the subtle properties of essential oils.

To make a very rich night treatment, suitable for those over forty

If you wish to make yourself a *very rich* night treatment, a face oil and/or an eye oil can be made using a vegetable oil as a base. Not all oils listed below can be used as a base or carrier, so I have included a percentage rating indicating the maximum amount that can be used for each individual oil. The "precious eye and mouth night oil" recipe given on page 102 produces truly amazing results. It is exciting to share them with you! I have tried many eye gels and creams and none of them come close to providing the moisturizing effect of this one.

Certain vegetable oils are best diluted into a base cream or another vegetable oil, as they are quite strong on their own. They are also a little more expensive (though very effective), so keep to the percentage described in the recipe. Some oils are edible, as indeed beauty comes from within. *Make sure that you buy cold-pressed vegetable oils only,* organic if you can, as it is going to be used on your skin.

Note: You need only to buy one or two oils to start with; the reason I name so many is simply to give you the best possible choice. If you are on a budget, buy something that you can use on your skin *and* eat as well.

LIST OF CARRIER/VEGETABLE OILS

Sweet almond oil (contains vitamins E, D, A, B1, B2, and B6) can be used as a base, 100 percent dilution.

Avocado oil (contains vitamins A, B1, B2, D, E) is very nourishing, great for dry skin; use only 10 to 20 percent in a base of your choice.

Borage/Starflower oil (contains GLA [gamma linoleic acid]) is good for those prone to thread veins, also for dry, "tired" skin and dry acne. Use 10 to 20 percent only in a base of your choice.

Carrot oil (rich in beta-carotene; also contains vitamins E, B, C, D) is rich in antioxidants, which makes it a great shield against damage caused by free radicals; also acts to slow down the aging of the skin. Use 10 to 20 percent in a base of your choice.

Evening primrose oil (contains GLA) is good for scar tissue, eczema, and psoriasis. It improves the skin's water-retaining abilities and helps to regenerate healthy cell membranes. Use 10 to 25 percent dilution in a base of your choice.

Hazelnut oil (contains vitamin E) is good for oily skin, irritated skin; it is absorbed very quickly. Use 10 to 80 percent in a base of your choice.

Linseed oil (contains omega oils 3 & 6) is good for irritated skin, dry skin. Use 10 to 80 percent in a base of your choice.

Macadamia nut oil is full of nutrients and is excellent to soften the skin, delay the aging process, and repair mature skin. Use 10 to 80 percent in a base of your choice.

Olive oil (contains vitamin E) is good for extremely dry, dull skin, scars, and stretch marks. It can also be used warmed up as a hair tonic. Use 10 to 80 percent in your base.

Safflower and sunflower oils (contains omega-6, vitamin E) are very affordable; good for dry, sensitive skin. Use 10 to 80 percent in your base.

Sesame oil (contains vitamin E)—I am talking about the cold-pressed oil here, not the toasted dark brown version that you can buy in most supermarkets. Sesame oil is water-soluble, so stains can be washed away. Although it filters about 30 percent of sunrays, it isn't strong enough to be used instead of a sunscreen, but it is certainly a very good oil to add to your base for a daytime moisturizer. Use 10 to 80 percent in your base.

Wheat germ oil (contains vitamins A, D; very high in vitamin E) is good for scarring, stretch marks, and aging skin. Do not use if you have wheat intolerance; choose instead avocado or any of the other oils named above.

***Jojoba** is technically *not an oil* but a liquid wax and is *not edible.* It leaves a film of protection on the skin and helps with moisture control. Jojoba has been a valid replacement in the cosmetic industry since the use of sperm whale oil has been prohibited by governments who have integrity. It is a very useful ingredient to add in your eye and mouth oil: it helps in reducing those thin "bleeding lines" around the mouth. Keep it out of the fridge, but store in a dry, cool place.

Tip: All those vegetable oils should be kept in a dry, dark, and cool place. Some of them, like linseed and hemp oils, should be kept in the fridge. If you buy a larger quantity of some of those oils and they are sold to you in a plastic container, transfer them to a glass bottle. Otherwise, with time and depending on the thickness of the containers, the plastic molecules will mix in with the vegetable oil, making it therapeutically useless, not so pleasant to use, and possibly harmful for those of you with very sensitive skin.

BASIC KNOWLEDGE ON ESSENTIAL OILS

Since we are essentially focusing on rejuvenating treatments, I will only name the oils useful for that purpose

The art of aromatherapy, however, is far-reaching and offers remedies that can contribute to the healing of many physical ailments and much more serious skin problems. Essential oils also work on a *subtle level*—reaching and altering energy levels—and are therefore useful in helping to heal deep emotional scars, assist spiritual healing, and deepen meditation and visualizations.

Note: If you are interested in the cosmetic and healing properties of essential oils, you will enjoy reading Patricia Davis's book, *Aromatherapy, an A-Z* (13) or *The Encyclopedia of Essential Oils* by Julia Lawless (20). For those of you interested in the use of essential oils in spiritual healing, read Patricia Davis's *Subtle Aromatherapy* (14).

All essential oils should be purchased from reputable sources *only*

This ensures that the oil has not been mixed or diluted, which would considerably lessen its therapeutic effect. Do not buy anything labeled "perfume oil" as they have nothing whatsoever to do with real essential oils. Synthetic perfume oils are toxic and have absolutely no therapeutic value. They might also cause serious skin irritation.

Precautions

Good-quality essential oils are obtained through steam distillation, solvent extraction, and expression, to name but a few. All these methods are intricate and require a lot of time and energy, which explains the cost of good, natural essential oils. Make sure that the oils you buy have not been exposed to direct strong light (neon, spotlight, or sunlight) as their potency would be greatly reduced.

Here are three more important tips:

- Reputable oils have their Latin names on the label, ensuring their provenance from a single botanical species.
- Buy them organic if you can, for a purer and stronger effect.
- *Essential oils should never be ingested.*

I have come across quite a few books with recommendations for internal use of essential oils. This is extremely worrying, as this is not safe at all under any circumstances. *Essential oils are very strong and have to be used with care.* They are highly volatile and therefore penetrate the skin within seconds; so there is *never* any need to ingest them for home usage.

If you would like to test that theory, put a small drop of lavender oil by your ear, and notice how long it takes for it to travel into your mouth and taste buds ... a fraction of a second!

REJUVENATING AND ANTI-AGING ESSENTIAL OILS

Damask rose (Rosa damascena) is very expensive but is one of the very best oils you can offer your skin. You need fewer drops of rose oil, as it is very powerful. It yields wonderful results on sensitive skin, broken capillaries, dry skin, and mature skin, and contributes to the prevention of wrinkles. The subtle properties of rose oil aid in the healing of deep emotional issues connected to the heart.

Note: If you come across rose oil that is very cheap (less than forty dollars for 5 ml), it isn't real rose essential oil. It takes a ton of petals to make a liter of rose essential oil, so it is expensive.

Frankincense (Boswellia carterii) has been used for thousands of years; our Egyptian ancestors knew of its properties and used it extensively for cosmetic preparations. Its preserving abilities are so efficient that it was also used for embalming bodies! It is also known and used as a tool for spiritual connection during meditating/praying. Good for young and mature skin alike, I is always better used as a preventative treatment: it is a very nourishing anti-wrinkle oil.

Neroli (Citrus aurantium bigaradia) helps the body to stimulate healthy new cells, which can delay the aging process by keeping the layers of connective tissue of the skin more elastic. Neroli is very good for mature skin, and is, just like rose, quite expensive, but well worth the investment. It can, like rose oil, be purchased in smaller amounts like 2.5 ml or 5 ml.

Helichrysum (Helichrysum angustifolium) is a more unusual oil. Also know as *immortelle,* it is another wonderful gift from Mother Nature. It helps to improve skin tone and delay the formation of wrinkles. It is good for young and mature skin alike.

Sandalwood (Santalum album) is a highly moisturizing oil. It makes a great addition to an aftershave cream, as it is also naturally cicatrizing and has a beautiful woody scent. Efficient when used on either greasy or dry skin, it has balancing properties and is useful in the prevention of wrinkles on younger skins. It has a beautifully masculine scent, which is what makes it so great in aftershave creams or lotions.

Ylang-Ylang (Cannaga odorata) is a sebum balancer, useful for those people who have combination skin. It has a deeply sensual and heady scent, and is often used as an aphrodisiac in massage oil. It is also thought to have antidepressant properties. It can be added to shampoo to stimulate hair growth (particularly if mixed with rosemary oil, providing you are not epileptic and do not have high blood pressure). It's good for younger skin.

Geranium (Pelargonium graveolens) is a very affordable oil and has properties that are similar to those of rose. This may be useful if you are on a budget and/or are still young and do not quite need rose oil yet. It is useful to prevent further broken capillaries; it also helps clear the complexion, re-establishes balance for combination skin, and helps to prevent wrinkles. It is greatly helpful for those of you who suffer from violent mood swings due to PMT.

Lavender (Lavendula latifolia/Lavendula angustifolia) is one of the greatest and most basic oils, definitely one to have around the house in a couple of different rooms, for emergencies: it is great used neat on kitchen burns (providing that the skin isn't broken; it is *one of the few oils that can be used without a carrier, for that purpose only*). It is used for many ailments such as acne, inflamed skin, sores and spots, and problem skin, and it is suitable for all skin types, as it has balancing qualities. It is an extremely safe oil and can be used diluted during pregnancy. A drop of lavender oil on your pillow can help you get to sleep; any more will keep you up.

Myrrh (Commiphora myrrha) is a more unusual oil. It has great moisturizing properties for very dry skin, although it should not be used during pregnancy. It is a powerful anti-wrinkle oil for mature skin and a useful tool for spiritual connection during prayer or meditation. Myrrh has been used since the beginning of time.

Benzoin (Styrax benzoin) is technically not an essential oil but a resin. It has a euphoric vanilla undertone and is, to my knowledge and experience, one of the most useful ingredients to moisturize super-dry skin on the hands and feet, extremely fast! It's best kept for hand and feet only, diluted in a base cream.

Note: Bathrooms are not a great place for oils, as these rooms are often too bright and too steamy; keeping them in a cupboard is slightly better, but another room is preferable.

LET'S MAKE THAT CREAM!

Okay, you now have the basic knowledge on the ingredients you need. Let me reassure you: you only need a few of them to make any particular cream. I give you several possibilities, so you can choose what you need, depending on your skin requirement and your budget. Before you start making your moisturizer, make sure that you have a glass jar because essential oils are strong and can work their way through plastic over time. Remember that this product is homemade and there are no added preservatives to extend its shelf life, so glass is a must, and using it within a six-month period will ensure its maximum strength. A colored glass jar would be even better to filter out strong light; you may be able to find those at the pharmacy, otherwise these can be found at essential oil stockists. If you can't find anything like that, just use an old jam or mustard glass jar, and simply keep it in a cupboard away from light and heat, with a label indicating what ingredients you have used.

"Fountain of Youth" moisturizer for women

This is designed as a powerful anti-aging cream for women thirty years old and over. You can start using it a few years earlier for prevention, using the oils recommended for younger skin; see the list of oils on pages 93-95. If you want a richer cream for a very mature skin, use a little more of the vegetable oils. If the recipe given below is too oily for you, use half teaspoons instead of full ones.

* Measures given are for a 60 g jar; adjust quantities according to jar size.

Fill a glass jar three-quarters full with Aqueous cream. Add:

One teaspoon of carrot oil (or wheat germ or avocado oil)
One teaspoon of evening primrose oil (or macadamia oil)
One teaspoon of jojoba oil (especially if making day cream)

Mix the base cream with the vegetable oils very well. It should not separate. If it does, you have put in too much vegetable oil; simply add a little more base cream to correct, and mix again until it binds.

Now you are ready to mix in your essential oils. Add:

Seven drops of rose essential oil (or neroli oil)
Six drops of frankincense oil (or myrrh oil)
Three drops of lavender oil
Mix all ingredients together; your blend is ready!

Optional: Add three drops of helichrysum essential oil for an extra anti-wrinkle treat—although it's not necessary, as the recipe given above will yield perfectly good results.

Put your blend aside until the next day. Rose essential oil needs time to "unfold"; there is precious alchemy at work in this beautiful pot of homemade cream you have just prepared. By morning, it will have blossomed and be ready to use. If you want to add a few extra drops of any essential oil, it is best to wait until the next day when all the scents have settled.

Note: If you want to make yourself a super-nourishing night product, simply swap the base cream with sweet almond oil. Follow the same instructions. At bedtime, you may want to cover your pillow with a small towel to avoid oil stains.

"Fountain of Youth" moisturizer for men

The same can be done for you gentlemen, and the product can also be used as a very effective aftershave treatment. The following cream is made with woody and green scents.

*Measures given are for a 60 g jar; adjust quantities according to jar size.

Fill your jar three-quarters full with Aqueous cream. Add:

One teaspoon of hazelnut oil (or wheat germ oil)
One teaspoon of linseed oil (or olive oil)
Mix the base with the vegetable oils thoroughly.

Now you are ready to mix in your essential oils. Add:

Four drops of lavender oil
Five drops of frankincense oil
Six drops of sandalwood oil

Mix all the ingredients together and you will have a very pleasing and extremely healing moisturizer/aftershave.

Note: Citrus oils such as lemon, lime, orange, or grapefruit may be added as long as there is no sun exposure after application. All citrus oils are photo-toxic, meaning that they disable the skin's natural defense against sun-ray damage.

Precious eye and mouth night oil

I have tried and tested many products that claim to moisturize the eye area and get rid of wrinkles, and I must say that I find them unsatisfactory for the most part. All of them disappear very quickly, leaving the skin very dry by morning. The following recipe will moisturize the skin to the point that it will still be supple when you wake up. We will be using base oils only, as *no essential oils* should be used around the eyes. Again, make sure you always use cold-pressed oils for best results, and organic whenever possible.

Use a nice small glass bottle, colored if possible

Colored glass is recommended for the same reason as for the cream. A brown medicine bottle is perfectly fine to hold this oil, although it will be nicer if it is a color that appeals to you—then all your senses are given a treat. I keep my eye oil in a beautiful blue bottle; I love this powerful rejuvenating potion as I know how well it works! You too will be nicely surprised if/when you try it.

*Measures given here are for a 100ml bottle; adjust accordingly if you are using a smaller/bigger bottle.

Fill a bottle a little more than halfway with almond oil. Add:

15 percent of borage oil,
15 percent of avocado oil, and
15 percent of evening primrose oil.

Put the top on and shake vigorously for a few seconds—that's it! Apply generously around the eyes and the mouth at nighttime; you will be pleasantly surprised by the results upon awakening.

Tip: Take it easy around the eye area when applying anything at all, as this skin is thin and very delicate. Starting with your right hand and your right eye, spread the oil clockwise. For the left eye, use your left hand and apply the oil counterclockwise.

Body lotion

To make a body lotion, you can use Aqueous cream or any of the other bases discussed on page 92. The idea is to thin out your cream so that it becomes fluid and therefore readily absorbable. You can use pure water, or even better some rose water—the same one we used to make toner.

For example:

1. To make a 200 ml bottle of body lotion, add about 50 ml of rose water to 150 g of Aqueous cream.
2. Mix those two ingredients thoroughly in a separate bowl. You can add more rose water if you want your lotion to be thinner.
3. Add in all the other oils as described in recipes page 100-101.

Tip: Use a little whisk, which you can buy from most kitchen shops, to mix your lotion; it is a miniature version of the utensil with which you beat your eggs. A fork will do just fine, though, if that is what you have at hand.

Toning and rejuvenating body lotion

I would like to give you a recipe for a body lotion that has toning and stimulating properties. The following oils will do wonders for promoting cell regeneration, and although they will not get rid of cellulite (as nothing applied topically can anyway … time for a reality check!), they will certainly stimulate blood circulation and therefore reduce congestion in those particular areas. This lotion will moisturize your skin, leaving it silky and fragrant, and while you are rubbing it in, you are effectively giving yourself a stimulating massage; which will assist your lymphatic system in the elimination of toxins (even better if you dry-skin-brushed before your shower).

Note: Some of the oils used can be very invigorating, so you might prefer to use this body lotion in the morning rather than at night. If you want to use it in the evening, omit the rosemary essential oil, as it may prevent you from sleeping. When you make your mixture, work promptly because the essential oils are very volatile and oxidize easily on prolonged contact with oxygen, thereby reducing their potency.

*Measures given here are for a 200 ml container.

Fill a large jar or a wide-neck bottle with your body lotion; I have used Aqueous cream diluted with rose water as previously described for the body lotion. Add:

One soupspoon of avocado oil

One soupspoon of wheat germ oil

Mix your base cream with the oils.

If you want something richer, you can increase the amount of oil a little, or add another such as olive, sweet almond, or rosehip.

Add the following essential oils:

Four drops of cypress

Three drops of rosemary (not to be used by people who suffer from epilepsy or by pregnant women)

Two drops of geranium

Two drops of ginger

Three drops of grapefruit/lemon or orange, as you prefer (or 1 of each)

Three drops of juniper

Three drops of sweet fennel

If you find this mixture too strong, reduce the amount of drops proportionally for best effect. If you would like it a little stronger, you can add one or two extra drops of each. Geranium oil can be quite overpowering, so be careful! If you find that your mix is too heavy with geranium (some droppers can pour very fast), use a few drops of lemon; it will disperse the heaviness of the blend.

MORE ESSENTIAL AND PRACTICAL TIPS FOR MEN AND WOMEN

DRY SKIN BRUSHING is extremely valuable to unclog the pores and get rid of accumulated dead skin cells, allowing the skin to breathe. It also gives a great boost to the blood circulation and the lymphatic system. Particular care should be taken to avoid the more fragile zones of the body and any areas with broken capillaries. You can purchase a good natural brush in most health food stores and some pharmacies; just make sure that the hair on the brush is of natural origin, such as cactus hair, hemp fiber, or something similar. Synthetic materials may cause skin irritation.

Method for dry skin brushing

All movements have to be done toward the heart to encourage the circulation to go with the natural flow. It also assists the lymphatic system to eliminate toxins from the body.

Tip: This may sound desperately obvious, but try to leave the brush where you can see it, so using it become a habitual gesture, as simple and as important as brushing your teeth! Your skin will be noticeably smoother with regular use and you will benefit from better blood circulation. This may contribute to keeping varicose veins at bay.

SHAVING can be a great source of irritation for the skin. Try using Aqueous cream instead of shaving foam for your legs, ladies, or for your face, gentlemen. It leaves the skin supple and moisturized. It is commonly used as a soap substitute by people who have serious skin conditions such as eczema and psoriasis.

A GREAT SOOTHING AFTERSHAVE can be made by simply adding a couple of drops of lavender oil to aloe vera pure gel. Aloe vera is packed with vitamins, minerals, and enzymes, making it useful for a wide array of complaints, both external and internal. For topical use only, the combination of aloe vera and lavender soothes irritated skin, as it has anti-inflammatory properties, stops bleeding (haemostatic), and disinfects the skin. Aloe vera also acts as a powerful anti-aging balm. It has many more uses, such as repairing and soothing sun-burned skin, superficial kitchen burns, etc. You might like to keep an aloe vera plant around and a tube of the fresh gel in the fridge for all emergency skin irritations.

EYE MAKEUP REMOVER is extremely harsh and too much rubbing around the eyes can contribute to broken capillaries, redness, and extra wrinkles in that sensitive and delicate area. I find the Aqueous cream extremely useful in its place. First, take off as much makeup as possible with a cotton wool pad soaked in water or rose water, then add a little cream on your pad and rub your makeup off gently. It leaves the skin clean, supple, and moisturized.

Note: The only time this won't work is if you are using waterproof mascara. Try using regular mascara as often as possible as the makeup remover used to take waterproof mascara off is very abrasive.

EYEBROWS give the eyes extra depth and definition when they look good, and make the face look younger. If you have a few white hairs in yours already, or simply want to have darker eyebrows, use an eyelash tinting kit and do your eyebrows every six weeks or so.

TOPICS EXPLORED IN SECTION 9

- Do you use a good moisturizer?
- Prevention and repair for beautiful skin
- Beauty thieves
- Golden tip for liver spots and skin rejuvenation
- Simple care for glowing skin
- Homemade recipe for anti-wrinkle creams, for men and women
- Extra practical and beautifying tips for men and women

NOTES

Chapter Two

FREE REJUVENATING SECRETS

1. The Tummy-Rubbing Exercise

LOSE INCHES FROM YOUR WAISTLINE … IN BED!

The Tummy-Rubbing exercise is extracted from Taoist philosophy

According to Taoist philosophy, the level of your wellbeing is largely reflected by the health and optimal functioning of your organs, which actually makes complete sense. There are many wonderful exercises in this rich tradition, but for now, we will explore one that is useful for the stomach, a source of unhappiness for many who carry superfluous weight or hold onto waste in that area. Before I describe this very simple exercise, let me remind you that we have dealt with the topic of food, its quality, and the quantity consumed on pages 1-5; and that *undereating of good nutrients* is one of the many secrets to staying young and healthy.

The following exercise is beneficial for:

- Efficient digestion after a large meal, acid stomach, flatulence
- Losing weight on the abdomen *and* all around the waist, otherwise known as love-handles
- Shedding localized weight rapidly after pregnancy
- Promoting regular bowel movements

So little work, so much benefit?

Yes, that's right! The fast results obtained by practicing this exercise are not magic, although it certainly seems like they are. What really takes place is *conscious assistance*. You are basically contributing to your own wellbeing by *physically* generating heat into your body and focusing on the desired outcome *mentally*. Your movements are precise and your intention is focused. Simple but powerful. The best place to do this exercise is ... in your bed! So don't even bother looking for excuses—you won't find any. Practice morning and night for fast and lasting results.

A really great secret that is over 6,000 years old

THE TUMMY-RUBBING EXERCISE

Physical movement

Rub your hands together, fast enough to generate heat.

1. Immediately place both hands flat on either side of your abdomen, one on each side.
2. Make circular motions, rubbing the abdomen with both hands simultaneously, starting from under your ribcage to just before your pubic bone. Looking down at your belly, your right hand is going clockwise and the left hand is going counterclockwise, similar to swimming strokes.
3. Keep your hands really flat so there is maximum contact and heat going into your abdomen. There is no need for strong pressure, and don't use any oil or cream, as this would slow down your movements.

Mental focus

Visualize your goal. Whether you need to work on regular elimination, or getting a smaller waistline, stay focused!

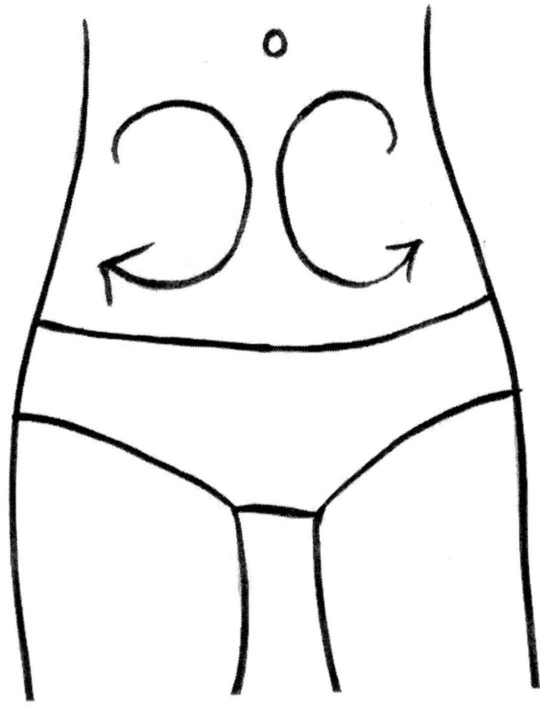

Tip: If you have difficulties with visualization, imagine cartoon characters like little fat cells leaving politely with a suitcase full of what you don't want!

STORIES FROM HAPPY TUMMY-RUBBING "USERS"

The end of beer belly

A student in one of my classes expressed his concern about his "beer belly" (his own words), so I shared this exercise with him. I explained the origin and purpose of the Tummy-Rubbing exercise and recommended he read Dr. T. Chang's book, *The Complete System of Self Healing* (11), for many more wonderful and easy-to-practice exercises. He decided to try it, although he admitted to being very skeptical. I should add at this point that he had a *sizeable abdomen,* with the rest of his body being of average built, a common occurrence when too much alcohol is consumed on a regular basis. He had tried various things, and although he had stopped drinking, nothing really worked to shed the weight from his stomach area. Having nothing to lose (but dead weight!), he started practicing the Tummy-Rubbing exercise and kept a detailed weekly report of the inches he lost. Within three months, he saw significant results and decided to come back and share his success with me. He reported being very surprised and delighted at the results this exercise produced, especially since it is so simple, relatively effortless, and definitely free of charge! A few months later, we met by chance in the street and his abdomen had completely *shrunk to a regular size*. He was absolutely delighted!

Reclaiming pre-pregnancy belly

I shed excess weight from around my tummy promptly after each of my three pregnancies using the same exercise. I never dieted once or deprived myself of the things I love. As I had many questions from women who took my classes, I included this exercise in my workshops. It is a secret definitely worth sharing, so pass it on to your friends and family. Anyone who has had more than one or two pregnancies knows that the challenge gets harder when it comes to regaining a reasonably flat stomach. Anyone over thirty-five who has trouble shedding weight around the abdomen will benefit by practicing this easy exercise.

Note: For further studies on self-healing exercises, read *The Complete System of Self Healing* by Dr. Chang. It is full of practical and self-empowering exercises for men and women.

TOPICS EXPLORED IN SECTION 1

- Getting rid of excess weight around the abdomen
- Improving digestion and elimination
- The Tummy Rubbing exercise

NOTES

2. Rejuvenating Exercises

A supple body makes for a supple mind

There are many fun and effective ways to keep your suppleness, energize your body, and lift your spirit. Yoga is one of the many ways possible to achieve greater health and balance in your life. It is accessible to all people, as most exercises are very easy and extremely gentle, regardless of your age or your physical condition.

Gentle exercises to awaken your Life Force

If you are young but "suffer"' from a lazy disposition, or are older and cannot consider joining a yoga class for whatever reason, you can do the following exercises from your bed in the morning.

Stretching is a great way to awaken the body gently, so make sure you follow the movements that your body wants to do; this is a good time to tune in and become aware of your presence in the room.

Yawning and humming gently opens up the throat and vocal cords; it generates a good vibration throughout your whole body-temple!

Smiling is great; always start the day with a smile. Smile at your partner, smile at your children when they come in, and smile at yourself when you meet in the mirror! Extend your smile down to each and every part of your body before you get out of bed; you will feel energized and much brighter.

Rotating your hands and feet can be done easily while lying down; it loosens your joints gently and stimulates good blood circulation for the day.

Gently move your head from side to side first (sitting up is best for this), then front to back. Repeat this several times until your spine, neck, and head feel "awake."

A NOTE ON GENERAL EXERCISING

Some exercises can do more harm than good

Imagine investing time, energy, and money to get fit, only to find that you have caused damage to yourself, and in fact, that you seem to have aged a few years ... yikes! For example, jogging along hard tarmac roads in busy cities not only stacks up the spine every time the feet touch the ground, but also seriously damages the lungs as they expand looking for extra oxygen, only to find carbon dioxide. Added to this, unless adequate sun protection is used, the skin can become seriously weather-beaten.

SAFE EXERCISES

Safe jogging

If you really like to jog, then running on soft ground, away from traffic is definitely a wiser choice. Make sure you wear adequate sunscreen and bring some water. If you can't be bothered to jog (I'm with you on that one; why run when you can walk?) and still want to do some easy outdoor exercise, then walking briskly is a really good option.

Brisk walks

Walking fast is very beneficial, as it speeds up the cardiovascular system. You can walk quite fast without having to do "the chicken walk," though there is certainly no harm in that aside from the funny factor! Choose an area that is free from too much pollution.

Cycling

This is also great and is relatively safe, depending where you cycle. You might consider making walking and cycling your mode of transportation, if at all possible, especially if you haven't got a lot of extra time for daily exercise. Again, make a plan to organize things in your life to accommodate exercise, rather than look for excuses, which does absolutely nothing good for your health or your self-esteem.

Swimming

This is an all-around pleasurable sport that benefits your whole body and is also very relaxing. All exercises done in the water are easier, as gravity is alleviated; it is a good option if you want to be particularly gentle on yourself.

Dancing

If you want to dance as a means to exercise, there are plenty of styles to choose from. Belly-dancing is great fun (and helpful for preparing to give birth, as was the original intent); dancing your emotions through the five rhythms (originally devised by Gabrielle Roth) can be very empowering. Or you could learn salsa, tango, ballet, ballroom dancing, and many more styles while having great fun, exercising, and making connections.

Slightly more adventurous but definitely good fun …

Pole dancing is now being taught as a mainstream exercise; it's a great rejuvenating practice because it puts you in an inverted position, which means fresh blood is circulating to the head and face. And it could spice up your conjugal life!

THE MOST AGE-DEFYING EXERCISES

If you are serious about doing yoga, Pilates, chi kong, tai chi, capoeira, or anything else that is new for you, I strongly recommend that you join with a group to begin with. Using tapes or DVDs at home is fine if you have already had some classes with a teacher; otherwise, you might injure yourself in the absence of any supervision. You also need *strong willpower* to keep up practice on your own at home, which also makes taking classes helpful. There are so many different types of classes available today; it is easy to find something you really like, and *passion fuels motivation*! Some exercises and practices are dynamic in nature, and some focus on stillness. Choose a mix of both for maximum benefit.

Tip: It is important to work on your inner core strength and muscle tone, particularly after the age of thirty-five. Remaining toned and supple while keeping excess weight at bay are among the physical challenges you face with the decision to age gracefully. Certain types of exercise focus on suppleness alone, which is not enough; be sure to include some gentle muscle toning in your routine, preferably something you will be able to keep practicing as time goes on. Pilates, for example, includes suppleness and gentle strength-building exercises.

A BASIC REJUVENATION POSTURE

Inverted postures are some of the most age-defying exercises

In these postures your body is upside down, literally. This allows the blood flow to circulate directly to the head, a rare occurrence. If you can do a head- or handstand, this is great! Be sure to include it in your daily exercising. *Do not take unnecessary risks: if this is not suitable for you, do not try it.* You can do one of the exercises offered below as an alternative; they are both extracted from yogic practice, and are safe and easy. Any posture in which your legs are raised above heart level will work on improving the blood circulation.

Caution: These postures are not suitable for people who suffer from high blood pressure and/or heart conditions.

Shoulder stand (A)

- Lie flat on your back, on the floor, feet together, with nothing under your head.
- Using your arms, elbows bent, raise your legs and back towards the ceiling.
- Your arms are supporting your back and help you to stabilize your position.
- Your back and legs are making a right angle with your head.
- Your chin is touching your chest.
- Stay focused and present through your breathing.
- Hold this position for anything from a few seconds to five minutes.
- Release your posture gently, making sure that your spine unravels slowly while making contact with the floor, vertebra by vertebra.

The plough (B)

If for some reasons you cannot do the shoulder stand exercise, you'll find the plough a gentler and easier version that is just as beneficial.

- Lie flat on your back on the floor, and raise your legs over your body, using your abdominal muscles.
- Use your hands to stabilize your position.
- Your legs are over your upper body; keep this posture for as long as is comfortably possible (or five minutes). If you are very supple, lower your legs behind your head until they are parallel with the floor; your feet can reach behind your head, touching the floor if possible.
- Stay focused and alert through your breathing.

Other benefits: These basic yoga postures help to promote blood circulation, contribute to clearing lung-related problems, tone legs and abdomen, and sharpen the mind. Have you ever seen small children tumble upside down on the sofa, especially when they have a cough or a cold? They know instinctively what to do to assist their own healing process.

Tip: If you cannot do either of these postures, simply raise both your legs above heart level while lying down. If you suffer from poor blood circulation, or have a stationary job where you cannot sit down, you will benefit by extending this practice to your bed. Simply put a few cushions under your mattress at the bottom of your bed—you will wake up feeling a whole lot lighter. See the Alexander Technique on pages 130-132.

THE SHOULDER STAND (A) THE PLOUGH (B)

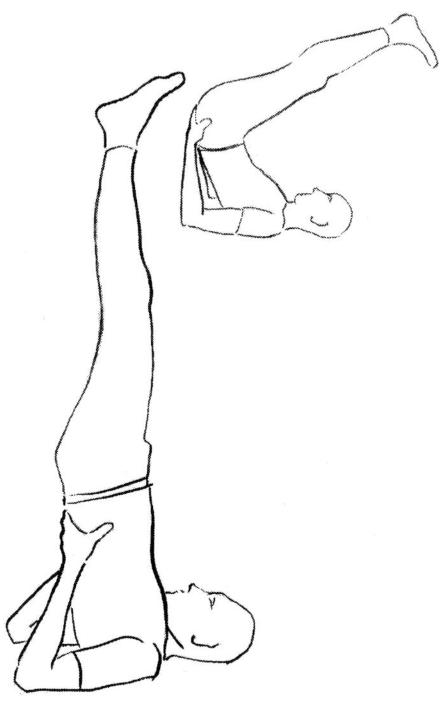

TRAMPOLINE

Bounce your problems away!

Bouncing on a trampoline a few minutes every day is a great way to give your cardiovascular system a good workout and stimulate your lymphatic system. I am not talking about an Olympic trampoline here, although if you have one, you and the kids will have great fun! You can buy a smaller version that is very affordable and is only inches from the ground so it can be used indoors. It is small enough so it can be lifted and put away if you live in a flat or have limited amount of space.

The use of trampoline is great for many things:

- It contributes to the elimination of toxins by stimulating the lymphatic system.
- It can promote bowel movements.
- It accelerates the removal of toxin overload while fasting (see page 147 for more information on detox methods).
- It is a good measure to find out if your PC muscle is in good condition (see below for explanation).
- It shakes and wakes the body up!

IS YOUR PC MUSCLE IN GOOD HEALTH?

The PC muscle is also known as the pelvic floor muscle (pubococcygeal muscle). Both men and women can find it when they try to stop urinating in mid-flow. Most of us tend to only become aware of certain parts of our anatomy when there is a problem, which is often too late, so better be pro-active!

Simple test to find out the state of your PC muscle

If you lose a little urine when you sneeze, laugh, cough, bounce, or run, you need to work on tightening up your PC muscle *urgently*, like right now as you read this. The longer you leave it, the harder it is to tone up and the more chances there are for serious problems to develop.

The PC muscle can be loose or damaged due to:

- Childbirth
- Excessive and repetitive sporting activities
- Strenuous pushing due to chronic constipation
- Aging
- A healthy PC muscle:
- Prevents instances of future incontinence
- Can prevent a prolapsed uterus, bladder, vagina, womb, or rectum
- Contributes to the ability to receive and give more pleasurable orgasms for both men and women, as it promotes better control of the vagina or penis
- Can help with easier childbirth and accelerate the healing process for postnatal recovery

Exercises for your PC muscle

They are called Kegel exercises and were named after Dr. Arnold Kegel, an American gynecologist. They are practiced with the aim of restoring the tone of the PC muscle and aid in the prevention of all related health issues as mentioned above.

The following exercises:

- Are very *easy to practice*; you *don't need to buy or use* any special equipment
- Can be practiced *absolutely anywhere*: while walking or sitting down, while traveling or working, etc.
- Can be practiced in series of ten or twenty movements, once or up to five times a day

Exercise 1: Squeeze your PC muscle, which is the same muscle you would use if you tried to stop urinating in mid-flow. Hold for three seconds and release.

Exercise 2: For example, in a set of ten squeezes, hold your PC muscle for ten seconds each time, and on the last squeeze, tighten your PC muscle as hard as you can before releasing altogether.

Note: The only challenge you face regarding the practice of these simple and beneficial exercises is to *remember to do them*. So maybe leave a discreet note around the house, the car, or the office that only *you* can understand; after all, PC also stands for personal computer!

Don't wait for a special time, or delay practicing them until you start a whole new routine—try it NOW while you read this!

HOUSEWORK

Housework might not be the most inspiring kind of workout, but it certainly has its place among exercises!

It is available to all of us and, unless your income allows you to employ someone to clean your house while you go and do some other kind of exercise; look at it as another opportunity to keep fit!

Stop complaining about it: Just do it!

There is no faster way to materialize those changes you have been waiting for in your life!

Things, events, and fresh energy can only come into your life if there is room for it. If your house is dirty and full of clutter, inquire within to see how you feel inside, what is really going on with you? Dirt and clutter affect all your layers: physical, emotional, mental, and spiritual. A house or a car very much reflects on your inner state; so think of that dirt and clutter as dead weight that is crowding your personal freedom and blocking the way for novelty to come into your life. Simply get to it, with friendly or paid help if you need to; you won't regret it. Stay focused and alert while you work your way through decluttering, don't let your memory of the past block your present actions—meaning don't hold onto those things (just in case …) when what you need to do is to get rid of them. Keep your intention firm and watch whatever you need most come into your life *effortlessly*!

Cleaning and tidying up are rituals

Cleaning and tidying up are essential and make complete sense when you think of them as *honoring yourself* and the space that *you live in*. Do it with as much joy and awareness as you would your daily exercises, meditation practice, prayer, or anything else that you do to honor yourself.

When you find the same contentment in cleaning toilets as you do in your spiritual practice, know that you have made a huge step on your path!

Tip: Why do it tomorrow when you can start today? Feel the difference in your body and your mind when you actually do something that needs doing NOW, versus putting it off. Putting it off adds a little extra weight to your thinking-load every time you remember it, only to have it sit at the "back of your head," increasing your mental clutter. Getting things done allows you to feel empowered, freer, and lighter!

Note: The cleaning products today are very strong and most of them are extremely toxic; they definitely contribute to damaging your skin and your lungs. You don't really need hundreds of sprays, cans, and bottles to do a good cleaning job. One or two simple products from the green brands are plenty around the house. A clean house is odor-free,—it doesn't have to smell of cleaning products.

TOPICS EXPLORED IN SECTION 2

- Simple bed exercises for all
- Body- and health-friendly exercises
- Age-defying exercises
- Bounce your problems away with a trampoline
- Keep fit inside-out with a healthy PC
- Ritualizing house chores to increase your life potential

NOTES

3. Laughing and Breathing

THE IMPORTANCE OF LAUGHTER

Laughing opens up and energizes the whole body

And it is absolutely FREE! There is something wonderful about laughter; not only does it release tension but it also uplifts your spirit. Laughing for fifteen minutes a day can contribute to your overall health: mental, emotional, and physical. It can contribute to the prevention and healing of certain cancers, in particular that of the throat. You can do it on your own (although not in a public place for obvious reasons!) or, better still, with a friend or two. It is completely safe and should be practiced as much and as often as possible.

Fake it 'til you make it!

If you have trouble laughing, start forcing yourself a little to begin with. I am talking about "belly laugh" here, so put your hands on your stomach to make sure you feel a vibration there too, not just in the throat area. If you don't feel any vibrations in your stomach area, practicing a few breathing exercises would be useful. If you are short of "funny friends," why not join a Laughter Yoga class? These courses are available worldwide by now; they are really good fun, as there is always someone there who has one of those "contagious" laughs, making it hard for even the grumpiest person not to join in! If there are no classes available in your area, why not start one? If all else fails, you can always watch a comedy!

BREATHING

Breathing is our most important "nutrient"

Thankfully, this mechanism is taken care of by our subconscious mind, so we don't have to remember to do it, or else we would all be dead! However, this does not necessarily mean that you breathe to your full capacity: stress, bad posture, blockages in the body, and smoking can all limit your ability to breathe fully. Shallow breathing further limits your well-being while depriving your cells of precious regenerating oxygen.

Restricted breathing shrinks your life potential accordingly.

Take a deep breath for an expansion of your potential

Notice what happens when you hear bad news or when you get into an argument? You almost stop breathing, your throat tightens, your whole body tenses up; you implode, explode, or freeze up. Your re-action is usually far from your potential. Taking a deep breath not only gives you a little time to process what is happening, but it also helps you to relax and gather your best resources to deal with the situation at hand, meaning that you can act with more awareness. In other words, becoming present, alert, or conscious enables you to proceed in the best possible way. *The trick is to remember to do it,* which may take a little training, but with a little bit of extra awareness, you can manage just fine. Whether you become alert first and then remember to take a breath, or take a deep breath which helps you to become alert, you are doing great! Remember: *Right action always comes out of presence.*

On a physical level, deeper breathing allows your cells to renew themselves to their fullest capacity. The amount and quality of oxygen received by your body also determines how much work your lymphatic system can accomplish. The lymphatic system facilitates the elimination of toxins present in your body. In short, breathing to your full capacity promotes better health on all levels. Take in as many deep breaths as you can, as it is one of the last natural resources that has not been harnessed for profit.

Simple breathing exercise

Find a quiet spot and sit comfortably straight. Leaning against a wall or the back of a chair is fine. You can lie down if you like. Closing your eyes might be helpful.

- Place you hands on your abdomen.
- Take a slow breath, deep enough that you can feel your hands rise as your diaphragm expands.
- Exhale slowly, at the same pace as your in-breath.
- Respect the natural pause between each inhalation and exhalation; simply allow your natural rhythm to play out.

Note: Before attempting to take a deep breath, it is important to ensure that you can do so: exhale all the air out of your lungs before inhaling. This allows the stale air to move out and make room for the fresh.

Tip: When in a confrontational situation, become centered by taking a deep breath. This will sharpen your focus and increase your response-ability. It could save the day at the office, on the road, before sharing your feelings with friends and family, etc.

TOPICS EXPLORED IN SECTION 3

- How much do you laugh every day?
- Learn to breathe fully for an expansion of your potential

NOTES

4. The Alexander Technique

The grace and benefit of good posture

Whether you are in your twenties or your seventies, male or female, one thing is sure: a bad posture is always unattractive. It takes away from natural poise as it cuts the person's presence. And it is often a source of back pain: it is literally as if years of troubles and worries are carried in a huge rucksack weighing the host down—an exhausting load that can be hard to drop.

The Alexander Technique raises body-awareness; subtle changes start to take place as physical patterns are shifted. In reality, the body has a natural yearning to realign itself according to its innate intelligence, and the Alexander Technique gently facilitates this process. Having regular sessions with your local practitioner is a wonderful investment in your well-being; you may even find yourself at ease in your own body for the first time in your life!

WHAT IS THE ALEXANDER TECHNIQUE?

Frederick Matthias Alexander was a Shakespearean actor (1869–1955) who lost his voice and could not be helped by the medical body. Based on a technique of self-observation, he researched and resolved his own problem within eight years. The Alexander Technique can be used as a powerful tool to help you become aware of how you inhabit your body and the space around you, and allow you to gain grace and ease while performing daily habitual movements. You can take individual lessons from a teacher but there is also a powerful and simple exercise you can practice safely at home by yourself.

The Alexander Technique can help to improve:

- Body mobility by making gestures more fluid
- Coordination

- Your sense of balance
- The way your body supports itself
- Your posture and natural poise

It enables the body to re-educate itself and facilitates the use of an *appropriate amount of effort* for any particular task. The result is that you have more energy at your disposal, as it isn't spent on holding up obsolete patterns. I must say that if you are on your personal quest to awaken, this technique offers valuable support to assist you in remaining or becoming alert throughout the day. This is a precious and easy tool anyone can use.

Personal experience

I find the Alexander Technique very useful and *extremely easy to practice*. There is no equipment involved in order to practice the exercise given below. If you can lie down with a book under your head, you can do this exercise. I have found it to be of great benefit, as it has helped me to correct my posture; it has contributed to the way I walk, how I position myself when I do some awkward DIY (Do-It-Yourself) around the house or while I sit down typing for long hours. It has helped the way I take in-breaths and best of all: I find myself inhabiting my body much more comfortably and with far more ease. The daily practice of this simple exercise has considerably reduced chronic back pains I used to experience and makes me more conscious about my body language in general.

Who can benefit from the Alexander Technique?

Learning about this technique can also be beneficial for a varied spectrum of professionals such as: public speakers, singers, actors, dancers, teachers, therapists, sports players, manual laborers, office workers, drivers, pregnant women, etc. It aims to eliminate the tension and stresses of everyday life by generating more awareness around movement and posture for all.

THE CONSTRUCTIVE REST POSITION

Let me share this wonderfully easy exercise with you. You can practice it every day, several times a day if you feel the need for it.

- Lie down on the floor with a book under your head. The book's thickness should allow your head to rest in a relaxed manner, which does not interfere with your breathing flow or push your chin into your chest.
- Fold your legs up so that your feet are flat on the ground, shoulder width apart, far enough from your bottom (as to not cut the blood circulation) and close enough so the abdominal muscles and the lower back are not strained.
- Your legs should feel relaxed, and their positioning should not incur any effort.
- Your back should touch the floor. If you find an area that does not make contact with the floor, simply become aware of it without trying to change it.
- Do not force anything; this may start to correct itself with regular lying-down sessions.
- Close your eyes, if you like, but stay alert.

Tip: For maximum benefit, remain in this position for 17.5 minutes, which is the total amount of time it takes for the intervertebral discs to come back to their normal shape and size. If you cannot stay lying down for so many minutes straight away, start with less, like five minutes or so, and increase the time with regular practice.

Another simple but powerful rejuvenating technique for your body

THE CONSTRUCTIVE REST POSITION

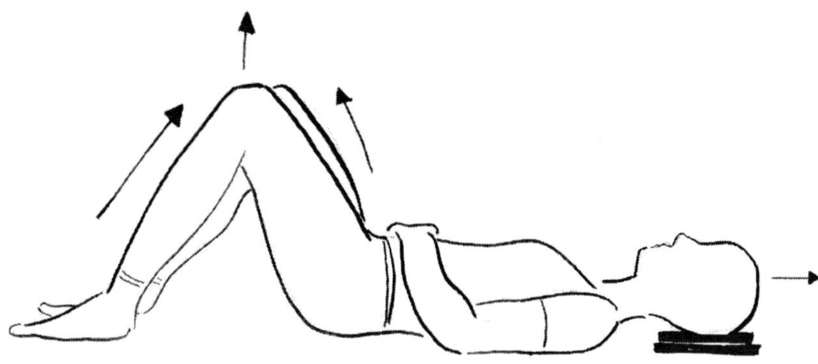

Note: You might already know that we go to bed a little shorter each night than we woke up. As we go about our daily activities, our whole spine gets compressed: the weight of the body puts pressure on the spinal discs, which effectively shortens the spine a little. Upon waking each morning, the discs between each vertebra have had a chance to regain their "springiness," so we wake up a little taller again. The Alexander Technique allows the body to regenerate itself in a very similar manner and can be done whenever necessary.

See Michael Gelb's book *Body Learning* (15) for more details on this practice.

TOPICS EXPLORED IN SECTION 4

- Are you conscious of your posture?
- Inhabit your body comfortably with the Alexander Technique
- Learn poise and grace through the Alexander Technique

NOTES

5. The Art of Challenge

DEALING WITH MENOPAUSE

Many women report "feeling invisible" while going through menopause

For some, going through this natural cycle can be a challenging experience, often rooted in negativity. This is due to several factors:

- Menopause is unfortunately nearly always perceived as *a disease* to be remedied rather than a natural cycle that needs support.
- There is a definite focus (or obsession?) in our society on younger people, particularly when it comes to women.
- Buying into one or both concepts above without challenging the beliefs that have been programmed into you!

Feeling invisible is among the hardest things to bear—yet who is in charge of this?

Let us not forget that concepts or people have power over you *only if you accept them.* If you give your power away, it is only reasonable to assume that it will be used, unfortunately probably against you. So let's look at the full picture.

Acknowledging some physical facts

At the onset of menopause, menstruation dries up, the skin begins to lose some of its elasticity, some extra weight can accumulate around the midriff area, hot flashes and various other symptoms can be experienced. Children want to live their own lives; some are actually leaving home. Your own parents may be experiencing serious health problems and you may need to take care of them. What a role reversal! All of those are factual possibilities that can become a source of emotional disruption, making this natural transition a hard time to bear for many women. There may be a lot of changes taking place, but then again, weren't there always?

Taking care of yourself is *primordial* and *not selfish*

You have to take care of your own needs. This has always been the case, but a sense of guilt may have prevented you from treating yourself in the way that you deserved until now. *Guilt* is one of the common denominators among many mothers, a belief that has turned into an emotional illness left over from years of parental and religious conditioning.

A few important reminders, just for you!

- You are no good to anyone unless you are in good form, so spending time on yourself is essential, *not selfish*.
- You need to feel nourished and at peace with yourself to be able to offer real support to others; charity starts with self and at home.
- You can contribute to others' fulfillment *once you feel fulfilled yourself*; otherwise you are like an empty vessel, making all the right gestures in complete emptiness.

Note: If you experience extreme resistance while reading this, simply observe your reactions and the mental dialog taking place. Do not take part—simply look, listen, and feel what is happening—remain the *silent witness*. Somewhere inside, *you know* that *you deserve* everything that life has to offer, so who is blocking that prosperity from coming in?

GOING THROUGH MENOPAUSE WITH EASE AND GRACE

A medical herbalist can give you a tailor-made prescription that will not only deal with your physical symptoms but also nurture your emotional capacity so you can go through this natural transition with ease and grace. There is a lot of emphasis on the physical symptoms when in fact the emotional body is where most of the impact is felt. Herbs can nurture the most subtle transitions of hormonal fluctuations and their accompanying emotional equivalent. Some people favor the use of allopathic drugs and prefer to consult their GP. The choice is entirely yours; just make sure that you are fully aware of all the possible side effects. Some herbs are compatible with hormonal treatments; check with your health-care specialist.

Note: Herbs also make an excellent gift of health for the whole family, or for anyone in need of a boost. For example, an herbal tonic taken in the spring and/or autumn will nurture the body's ability to acclimate to the energy depletion resulting from the change of season, or any other challenges that take a toll on one's health.

Useful herbs for the varied symptoms of the menopause

If you cannot go to an herbalist, you can choose from many good herbs available over the counter at health food stores. You may need to change the herbs you take every few months if your symptoms come back, as your body can get "complacent" when treated with the same herbs continuously. Ask the store's qualified staff for what would best suit your particular requirements. While this may not be quite as good as a tailor-made treatment, it will certainly help a great deal, and many people find that they can get satisfactory results.

Choose from:

Wild yam
Red clover
Agnus castus
Dong quai
Black cohosh

The positive aspects of menopause

How about challenging the limiting beliefs that have been imposed on you? A shift of attitude is the most important ingredient for a gracious transition. While there are some undeniable biological changes taking place, your potential for maturity and wisdom is magnified. Inner beauty, which cannot be bought anywhere, is yours to unravel!

Positive attributes associated with this natural cycle:

- The kids are gone (or going soon), so you now have the time to do or study what you have always wanted, without those guilty feelings!
- It is time to reinvent yourself (hair, makeup, clothes?); after all, who cares what people think?
- By the time your menstruation stops, other more subtle spiritual energies come into play and you can access *your* most powerful female energy yet.
- Sexuality certainly doesn't have to stop; this is up to you. Connections are deeper and more meaningful, and the capacity for gratitude increases as you realize the transitory nature of this life you are living. If you truly realize this and can share it with your partner, you are in for an unforgettable time!
- Wisdom is powerfully beautiful. The fresh innocence of youth is replaced by magnetic attraction in women and men who have reached a certain level of experience and maturity ... something to be celebrated!

So rejoice, celebrate, and invite your wiser self to shine out into the world!

Note: If you are experiencing some difficulties about accepting the fact that your children are leaving home, understand that you have identified with your role as a mother/father. The time has come for you *to reclaim your identity*. Take some time for yourself and start by listing things that you *love* doing, or *would love* to do. Do not censor what seems to be out of reach for now; all achievements begin with a simple vision.

RETIREMENT ... DO YOU HAVE A CHOICE?

There are two kinds of retirement

The cessation of work and the decision to give up: they certainly do not have to go hand in hand. The *structural retirement* from your former employment does not have to become an *emotional retirement*. The first is a fact; the second is a *personal decision*.

Retirement from employment

This experience can be crushing for some people and can, in some extreme cases, lead to feelings of wanting to retire from life in general and sometimes to depression or other emotional illnesses. Yet for others, it can be a liberating experience.

The way that you experience this new challenge very much depends on your personal values and your belief system, which make up your perception. A tool to help you go through with this enormous change in your life is *acceptance* of the situation at hand. Any kind of inner resistance to this (whether you are about to retire or already have) will foster resentment, anger, and bitterness—in short, all the negative qualities that contribute to aging you a few more years and reducing your joie de vivre. See the Is-ness exercise on page 143.

It is undeniable that retirement can be challenge

It can bring up questions of self-worth, especially if you have spent most of your time working and dedicated your life to a particular profession. You have identified with your career and have lived your whole life through this lens. It is time to broaden your horizon. The first thing is to *not give up on yourself*. The second is to *not give in to the pre-arranged plan* that society has formatted for you. You may have been asked to retire but that does not mean that it should dictate your emotional attitude. Who wants to be boxed up and labeled as "non-recyclable" material? Yes, it is true that we live in a world largely made up of disposable commodities and that vibrant youth is favored over staying power, wisdom, and experience. So let us put this to good use by harnessing those facts and *turn this apparent adversity into our own strength.* The first and foremost work to be done is to eliminate negative beliefs.

CHALLENGE: A SECRET THAT KEEPS YOU FOREVER-YOUNG

Challenging yourself is one of the best things you can do to keep enjoying your life. If you haven't dared to dream *free enough* or *big enough* until today: now is the time! Close your eyes, open your imagination, and see for yourself *what you are truly capable of.* The older we get, the shorter the journey becomes, so why not accept everything that life has to offer? The process of opening up to new possibilities and trying things out is great fun; the outcome, in reality, is of no particular importance. Great things will certainly happen, but enjoying the journey moment by moment is the key to peace and well-being. This, by the way, needn't exclusively apply to retiring citizens: all ages are welcome! A challenge does not have to be an insurmountable task—it can be a simple dream you have not felt *free enough* to allow to take place in your reality until now.

It could be something very simple such as:

- Improving a relationship you have with a loved one (you may be the first one on the list)
- Letting go of the things from the past you wish you could change: you cannot—they've already happened. It is time you made peace with them!

- Learning something new like painting, wine tasting, tango, etc.
- Going back to college or university
- Writing that novel you so often talked about (who cares if it gets published!)
- Mentoring younger people from your area of expertise
- Traveling
- Keeping or developing an open mind: an open mind means a supple body (this prevents serious calcification of bones, as in arthritis)

In short, keep actively doing what you love most, or find new things that you can *feel passionate* about. Passion is one of the best anti-aging secrets.

A shift in attitude can be a catalyst for a shift in consciousness

In Native American tribes, for example, the Elders hold a very special place. They are respected and, in fact, revered by their younger peers for their wisdom and life experience; may this example inspire a shift in our society! Things are not going to change until you take a step in the direction of renewal. Each individual has personal wisdom he or she can share: all were young once and helped to build the foundations on which we live today. Check out my You Tube Channel (Mahayana Agent of Change) for a rejuvenating talk on The Elders.

Are you far away from retirement age?

Do not think that you are too young to contribute to this shift in consciousness *now*. The creative potential of "tomorrow" is in direct proportion to the widening of your perception today. Do not be afraid to contribute anything you can in any way possible; change usually happens in the minority of ONE. *Younger generations may choose to keep an open attitude toward their Elders and Elders need not succumb to their expected fate.*

Do you feel too small to make a difference?

Visualize this: *A huge room full of people. In comes a mouse ...*

Watch out for self-fulfilling prophecies

The power of self-fulfilling prophecies should not be underestimated: negative statements are just as powerful as positive ones, especially if they are used on a repetitive basis and with enough emotion fuel to make them materialize. Start by observing your main stream of thought and see where you need to inject some positive energy; or simply drop negative beliefs. Some of you in your sixties feel more vibrant and positive than when you were in your thirties. Never *sell yourself short*; whatever your condition or your ability, there is *something you can do* if you open your mind to it. There are many things you can share with the rest of the world—what are they? *Do not settle for what has been programmed into you; go for it—fulfill your potential!*

Creativity exercise

If you feel the need to channel your energy into something but are not quite sure of the direction, you may find this exercise helpful:

1. Take a deep breath, bringing your attention to your body and relax (a cup of tea or a glass of wine may be helpful here).
2. Start by listing all the things that you are grateful for. This could be skills, state of health, physical ability, awareness level, generosity toward self and others, support that surrounds you, etc.—anything that comes to mind!
3. Take an overview of the information before you, almost as if it were someone else's. If nothing comes to you now, leave the list aside and come back to it later. The idea behind this is to *stay out of your own way*, to let the *creative spirit move through you*.
4. Simply let inspiration crystallize into ideas; write freely, without censoring yourself.

Tip: If you find that "automatic blocks" or negative self-talk pops up when you begin to feel inspired, simply observe your thought mechanism without taking part. Stay present—do not contribute to it; it will pass.

Alternatively, you might benefit from getting help from a friend or even from someone a little less familiar, like a coach. A coach can often have a clearer perspective on the information given, as long as he or she refrains from judgment and personal opinions.

What to do if you do not feel pulled toward anything in particular

If you don't know what to do, that is absolutely fine—*do nothing*! Wait until you feel inspired because contrary to what you have been taught, *being* is always more important than *doing*. Surrender to the present moment and its simplicity, to the is-ness of your existence; and enjoy the peace that naturally flows from such a state of acceptance. Enjoy the following.

Note: Anyone wishing to challenge themselves will enjoy Jack Canfield's book, *The Success Principles* (9). Additionally, many heartwarming stories can be found in *Chicken Soup for the Soul* by the same author.

The Is-ness exercise

1. Find a comfortable place to sit or lie down, in any way you wish and anywhere you like.
2. Take a few deep, gentle breaths.
3. Notice your own presence by simply observing yourself: feel your body making contact with the bed or the chair, note your breathing rhythm, or pay attention to any sensations in your inner body
4. Gently say:

- I accept my life as it is *now.*
- I surrender to the *is-ness* of my existence.
- Things are perfect just the way they are.
- I am grateful to be able to observe this *now* and enjoy the simplicity of *being.*

You may find yourself physically smiling as you speak the last line. Let your smile expand and fill all parts of your body; feel its illuminating and healing qualities radiate deep joy, strength, and peace within you. If you find this exercise useful, you may extend it by letting your smiling energy permeate people and events in your life; ultimately, nothing is so serious in life that it should rob you of your peace of mind, only *you* can do that to yourself. Notice how much easier things appear to be, or how you feel next time you meet those people whom you formerly dreaded meeting. Simply observe without judgment or ownership.

For more self-awareness exercises, see Chapter Three.

THE ULTIMATE JOURNEY

Living life to the fullest

We all share similar challenges, with similar outcomes, one of them being that death is an ordinary process in our evolution. It is a fact that *tomorrow is promised to nobody,* so developing an ease about living is necessary. And it can be deeply gratifying. There is tremendous fear around this natural cycle in Western society, which is not surprising, since the dying or terminally ill are segregated away for none to see. This inhibits an otherwise natural human ability to understand and accept that *all forms are transient.* We tend to fear what we do not see. This, coupled with ominous predictions from various religious traditions, make impeding death a focus of fear and anticipation: the most perfect peace repellent! Being denied the experience of contact with death effectively blocks the way for the simple realization that *life, like all things, is transient and is a gift to be grateful for,* no matter what shape it takes. A large part of being at peace with yourself is to know that you have enough courage to try new approaches and to get up and move on when they don't work out in the way that you intended. Who cares? The fun is in the journey—not the destination—is it not?

For some people, however, a near-fatal encounter or the proximity of the end of their physical journey can have a freeing effect. The fear of death dissolves as the transition into non-physicality; it is experienced as a luminous process, or a sudden awakening. Daily life is then experienced as *fulfilling and joyful,* which was always the case, of course, but was not previously perceived as such due to lack of information, awareness, or a resistance to *simply being*. One day, when the time will have come for you to leave your present form, the quality of your physical departure will depend on your state of awareness. Realize that there is *no past* and *no future;* anything that ever took place or that will ever take place will always happen in the present, the *eternal now*. Ultimately, we all want to be at peace and have no regrets ... doesn't that sound like a fine recipe for life? Why not start living each day as if it were your last... .

This is undoubtedly the best kept secret to staying forever young!

TOPICS EXPLORED IN SECTION 5

- Redefining the transitional time of your life
- Menopause: new life cycle, fresh possibilities!
- Retirement on your own terms
- The creativity exercise
- The Is-ness exercise & the simple joy of being
- Living life to the fullest

NOTES

6. Detoxifying Methods

Detoxification is a huge contributor to superb health and rejuvenation

The following may sound a little mechanical, but would you expect your car to keep running without ever getting it serviced? No? Well, the same goes for your body. How can you hope for radiating health and rejuvenation while giving your body absolutely no support? It really is as simple as that.

There are some easy ways to detoxify your body and some slightly more challenging rituals that can take more time, more commitment, and more effort. All of them are extremely helpful and will help you to look much younger than your years, feeling fully regenerated upon completion. Not all the methods shared below are for everyone, so you might need to get professional advice and adequate supervision, *especially if you have health issues.* A handful of people report feeling unwell and suffering side effects after a basic detoxification, so do absolutely check with your health practitioner before undertaking any of the following methods. Remember that fear alone will bring on unsettling feelings, so make sure you do enough research before going ahead with anything discussed in this chapter. Once you have information and take a few moments to get a sense of what feels right for you, you are ultimately your own best guide!

Note: None of the following cleansing methods are intended for children or teenagers, pregnant women, or very elderly people. Wheat and sugar abstinence mentioned below, however, can benefit most people.

THE "EASY" DETOXIFYING METHODS

There are all sorts of easy methods to detoxify your body

- One can simply be giving up sugar- and wheat-based products for two or three weeks. This will greatly contribute to making you feel a lot healthier, very rapidly. It may give you an incentive to try something a little more daring, like fasting, for example (see page 154 for information on fasting).
- Giving up alcohol and cigarettes for a while can also be a great boost. If you think you have an "addictive personality," try this: feeling good is also addictive! By the time you feel healthier and lighter, have more energy, notice that your skin and your eyes are clearer (and have people comment on it so you know it's real!), you might consider altering your daily habits permanently.
- All sort of detoxifying products are available from health food stores and pharmacists. There are even detox-pads that you can stick under your feet at night, made from a mixture of crystals and essential oils. They work on drawing out toxins from your body through the soles of the feet, and are based on knowledge from reflexology, crystal healing, and aromatherapy. I find that they all work a lot better if you assist the process by also taking care of your lifestyle.
- Why not simply integrate some homemade fruit and vegetable juice in your daily diet? Any of the tips offered so far would be a plus. Certain herbs and foods are valuable assets to nourish, support, and help clear out your whole system.

LIST OF HERBS AND FOODS TO SUPPORT RADIANT HEALTH

Practicing prevention is always a wiser choice than relying on a cure. This can be used all year round as supporting care for your body, which is constantly at your service and works so hard for you! The herbs and vegetables named below can be used as specified to make tea and juices or to be eaten raw (or steamed as a last resort). *Remember that food is medicine for your body.*

For the liver:

An extra intake of bitter food is very toning, detoxifying, and strengthening for the liver:

Apple juice (homemade is best!)
Artichoke hearts or artichokes
Asparagus
Chicory salad
Dandelion salad
Dandelion coffee
Lemon juice (squeezed into a glass of water, with no added sweetener of any kind)
Milk Thistle
Yarrow tea

For the lungs:

Cayenne pepper (a pinch in an herbal tea or a dish; don't cook it, just add it before eating)
Comfrey tea
Basil tea
Rosemary tea
Seaweed as a food or in a bath (Carrigeen moss is great)
Thyme tea

For the kidneys:

Chamomile tea
Celery (tea as celery seeds or juice from the vegetable)
Cucumber juice
Dandelion tea or coffee
Fennel tea
Homemade barley water
Horsetail tea
Nettle tea
Onion juice

For the lymphatic system:

Ginger root for tea or grated in casseroles
Ginger bath (see method on page 153)
Cayenne pepper (see recommendation above for lungs)
Garlic and onion juice (or raw, mixed into a salad)
Beetroot juice

For the skin:

We have explored many different options to improve and rejuvenate your skin in sections in Chapter One.

Here are some more:

Carrot juice (20 percent mixed with another vegetable juice is plenty, as it is high in sugar)

Cabbage juice, red and green (brilliant for overall health and skin)

Cucumber juice
Fennel juice
Parsley tea (and raw herb)
Spinach juice
Sage tea (a "must" for superb health and rejuvenation)
Watercress juice

For the bowels: See page 66.

Note: Many of the fruits and vegetables 'cross-over' as some of them share similar healing and detoxifying properties. Juices are a wonderful thing to include in your daily routine; they are an *easy way* to consume your raw fruits and vegetables. The vitamins, minerals and enzymes are at their most potent when absorbed in this way, as there is no heat involved. This is a sure and easy way to alkalinize your body, and a fantastic way to prevent many serious illnesses and diseases.

See *Healing Drinks* by Anne McIntyre (22).

Fruit and vegetable juice recipe

This is my own recipe. It yields about one pint of juice and is wonderful before lunch or any heavy protein meal. Add or omit ingredients as you prefer. Buy organic produce if you can.

You need:

One carrot
Three stalks of celery
One apple
One-half a cucumber
One inch of fresh ginger root
One clove of garlic.

Juice all the above, and add the juice of half a lemon to it. Drink immediately for maximum freshness.

To your health!

DETOXIFYING BEAUTY BATHS

Detoxifying baths are a wonderful bonus to your health

Here are three different methods. They all have slightly different properties and are all powerful even if used on their own, but always better if used as part of a detox. *Don't forget to drink a glass of water before, during, and after any of these baths, as this will help your lymphatic system to eliminate toxins.* A candlelit room is always a treat and adds to the relaxing effect. This is a great time to visualize the *new you* and dream about your very bright future. Enjoy!

SEAWEED BATH: Most health food stores sell seaweed in its natural state or in powder form. Here in Ireland we are blessed to be able to get it directly from the sea in the autumn, when it is at its most potent with healing properties. Kelp and dulse can be used in equal amounts for one bath. Whether you buy the dried seaweed prepacked in a net or have dried your own seaweed at home, it needs a little preparation before adding it to your bath:

1. Boil some water and pour it over the seaweed in a separate pot or bucket. Steep in the boiling water for ten to fifteen minutes and pour it into your bath water. You may want to use the rest of the seaweed in the net as a "loofah" to rub onto your skin—a very nourishing treat!
2. If you are using the powdered stuff, put a very generous handful in your tub while the hot water is running.

The iodine released is wonderful and, with closed eyes and a little imagination, you could be at the seaside! Not only does it detoxify the body, but it is also packed with essential vitamins and precious minerals. It is particularly high in vitamin A, which makes it a *super-powerful rejuvenating treatment for the skin.*

Tip: You will maximize the absorption of vitamins and minerals if you remember to use dry-skin brushing before taking your seaweed bath. This is the closest thing you'll get to a spa at home—a great gift to yourself!

GINGER BATH: This has a very relaxing effect on the body. It also has deeply cleansing properties, which materialize as profuse sweating after the bath. Make sure you keep very warm to assist the process.

1. Simply grate the equivalent of about two inches of fresh ginger root and throw into your bath while the water is running. Make it as hot as you can reasonably bear. (Use the thinner side of a cheese grater for the ginger to best liberate the oils.)
2. Soak in the bath for about thirty to forty-five minutes.

Tip: If you are planning on going to bed straight after the bath, put a towel under you to keep your mattress dry.

HEAVY METAL DETOX BATH: This helps the body to rid itself of all unwanted toxic metals such as aluminum and mercury.

1. To running hot water add:
   One-half cup (125 ml) of bread soda (bicarbonate of soda)
   One-half cup of Epsom salts
   One-half cup of natural sea salt (unrefined if possible)
2. Soak in the bath for a minimum of twenty minutes for best results.

Note: What you will see is rather fascinating; the water will turn slightly murky brown as metals leave the body—better out than in!

THE "HARD" DETOXIFYING METHODS

Do you wake up easily, feeling light and full of energy? I mean enough energy to feel like you could kick the ceiling? No? Then have a look at the following detoxification recipes to see if you would like to try some of them. Some are "hard" in the sense that they take more commitment and a little more time to achieve, but they are all wonderfully effective; you will be able to *see and feel* the benefits within days of completion. This is rejuvenation you can physically appreciate; *you will feel and look like you have lost ten years*!

FASTING

A note of caution before we explore different methods of fasting

I am solely talking about fasting for the purpose of detoxifying and healing the body right here. I am not talking about religious fasting, or fasting to lose weight. If you fast with the intention of losing weight, you are wasting your valuable time, as I assure you that you will regain every ounce you lost, possibly with a few on top. Fasting was never meant as a way to get slim. Children and teenagers *should not fast under any circumstances*; their bodies are developing and therefore need regular and healthy nutrients.

What is fasting?

Fasting consists of the abstinence of food in order to allow the body to self-regulate and repair itself. Fasting can also be of tremendous benefit as a means to maximize the body's natural self-healing capacity when faced with very serious physical illness, but this requires supervision from a health professional. We are only exploring fasting for its self-rejuvenating properties in this book.

The decision to fast, whether made by instinct or intelligence, has been followed in nature by all beings since we came into existence. It is practiced to assist an organism in ridding itself of toxic overload and viruses, thereby freeing itself from pain, disease, and discomfort. All animals fast instinctively when unwell. Fasting is one of the most ancient rituals used for allowing the body to regenerate itself on all levels, including the spiritual. While the body is freed from processing the food usually eaten, its innate intelligence works without interruptions to repair the body. This is why it is often better not to eat while illness is present; juices, herbal teas, and of course water can be taken instead of food.

The physical benefits of fasting

Fasting clears clutter from the physical body and, as a result, purifies the mind, as both are intrinsically linked. It has proved useful, in some cases, as a method to end years of chronic depression. After several fasting periods, you may witness the elimination of the black lining, also known as mucoid plaque, which usually coats the colon and is made up of sticky waste. This lining has been accumulating since childhood and is responsible for keeping a high level of toxicity in the colon. Having been accumulating progressively for so long, it does not shift easily. No wonder those "black moods" remain, even after so many years of counseling or various other therapies. *It is incredible to realize that we can hold so much poison in our body, and powerful to understand that it can be cleansed naturally.*

As previously mentioned, research shows that chronic constipation can, in some cases, contribute to the proliferation of certain cancers in the colon, prostate, womb, etc. Fasting cleanses the colon thoroughly and naturally, so invasive methods such as colonic irrigation are not necessary to achieve results. In fact, colonic irrigation does not deal with the elimination of mucoid plaque at all. Fasting is a powerful tool to prevent diseases, premature aging, and death in some extreme cases (see the book recommended below).

Note: Read *The Breuss Cancer Cure* by Rudolph Breuss (7) for some very interesting research on the healing of cancer.

For the fastest and easiest way to eliminate mucoid plaque, go to www.blessedherbs.com, where you can buy readymade fasting kits.

The subtle benefits of fasting

Fasting amplifies your awareness, refines the senses, and redefines the aptitude to make better choices according to your instinctive abilities. All your senses are enhanced while you are fasting, as you are getting rid of many toxic layers; you can smell, see, and feel things like never before. It can certainly be very helpful if you are trying to make a clean break toward a healthier lifestyle, or if you are going through a major transition in your life. For example, if you would like to get rid of an addiction to alcohol or nicotine, fasting can facilitate a clean break while the necessary changes are put in place.

The Herxheimer reaction is another name for a healing crisis in which a large amount of toxins are being released into the body, in this case brought on by fasting. These symptoms can include headaches, joint pains, and fatigue almost assuredly for everyone, as the body is working to push out unwanted toxins. Vomiting, diarrhea, and irritability are less common but may occur as a result of the body going through self-cleansing. This is why some people give up the fast, thinking that they are getting sick, when in fact the body is just beginning to cleanse itself deeply. It helps to have the support from someone with previous fasting experience while you try this method for the first time.

Fear of fasting?

The fear of fasting is common in our Western society; it is essentially based on a lack of knowledge. Once you have read enough information (and/or talked to people who have fasted) and you feel comfortable enough to start a fast, choose carefully with whom you surround yourself at that time. Some people may have a negative impact on you, especially if you are easily influenced, as they may not understand your choice. Although their fears are solely based on a lack of information, they may destabilize you if you are feeling a little vulnerable. You need love and support, not fear and worry-energy. Find a comfortable and safe place while you are going through your cleansing ritual—look at it like a retreat. If you are living with friends or family, explain to them what you are doing clearly so they don't start worrying unnecessarily and trying to feed you constantly!

Fasting can be an amazing experience

The benefits of fasting are visible soon after completion, which will give you another great boost. The whites of your eyes clear up due to the liver being regenerated, your skin is glowing, your hair is shiny, and eating is such an orgasmic experience that you'll never again look at food or eat it without true gratitude!

Helpful facts and tips:

- You can get quite cold while you fast, so make sure you wrap up warm. For the same reason, I feel that fasting is best done in the spring or summer, which is also most conducive to regeneration.
- Some people believe that staying in bed is important while you fast, and some prefer to move around. I would agree with the latter. Moving around helps the lymphatic system to expel the overload of toxins.
- Bouncing on a trampoline for five minutes, several times a day, can be helpful to eliminating the nauseous feeling and headaches that may occur within the first two days of your fast. It stimulates the lymphatic system to carry out toxins, and you will feel an immediate relief. Nearly any

sport that you usually practice is okay; just see how you feel and do take it a little easier than usual.

- Drink PLENTY of water.
- If you are going to stay at home, keep active. This will take the focus off the fact that you are not eating. It is surprising to realize how much time and energy is spent on feeding ourselves once the activity is stopped!
- Why not do a "spring cleaning" at home while you fast? It is good to see that your home environment matches the inner renewal taking place. You don't have to move furniture around; you might simply tidy up some paperwork.
- Some people carry on working as usual. If you operate machinery, do stay very present. Ideally it would be better to take a few days off, but that isn't always possible.
- If you are working with food, then the challenge is all the greater. See how firm your will power is ... !

Preparation before a fast

Take it easy for a few days before embarking on a fast. Here are a few suggestions to make your journey smoother:

- Start by reducing the *big intake* of toxicity (e.g., don't start fasting the day after binge drinking)
- Reduce your sugar, tea, and coffee intake to one cup per day for two or three days before you start.
- Stop smoking. If you don't think you can quit for a few days, then don't fast. Absorbing poisons while trying to get rid of them is pointless!
- Set your mind on a preferred amount of days; whatever you choose is fine. You will find that once you make the decision clearly, it will be easy to keep to it.
- Fasting for two or three days for the first time is enough; you can do four or five days next time. One fast per year is enough.

- Stop taking vitamins or herbal treatments; your body is repairing itself and needs as little interference as possible.

Note: Some people like to fast just one day every week. While this gives a small break to the digestive system, it does not allow the body time to detoxify itself. Deep cleansing usually begins on the third or fourth day of your fast, so you may suffer the heavy headache of the first day with no real regenerative or detoxifying results.

Contra-indications to fasting

If you are on medication, consult a qualified practitioner before doing anything like fasting, as it may not be suitable for you. Do not fast if you are underweight or pregnant: just concentrate on eating vibrant and natural nutrients.

Emotional cleanse

Fasting is a good time to get rid of what you have been carrying in the way of emotional luggage. Writing a letter is a very good activity; you can write to someone who is here, someone who has passed on, or even someone with whom you are no longer in contact. The aim is to help you expel the emotional poison that you are holding onto. You can afford to express yourself completely freely, as you are not going to send this letter, but in fact burn it. This is a powerful ritual. The flames of the candle will devour your words and carry the energy back into the ether, freeing you from unwanted toxic burdens. You can start to feel the peace within you more clearly as the obstacles to your well-being are removed.

Note: This is a useful practice, whether you are fasting or not. Look within to see *who* you have been giving your power away to and write to them today. In some cases several letters may need to be written, depending on the severity of the person's grip on you. Remember to burn the letter!

DIFFERENT METHODS OF FASTING

The importance of enzymes

Enzymes not only assist the digestive process but also help in the natural elimination of toxins. They work in conjunction with vitamins and minerals by supporting and cleansing your metabolism. Fasting with raw fruits and vegetables can contribute to vibrant health as these foods are packed with enzymes in their original state.

Tip: Eating a piece of fresh pineapple or papaya facilitates the digestion of animal protein. This is due to the high content of enzymes found in both fruits.

A MONO-FAST is a one in which you eat one type of fruit, *only*. Say you choose apples; you can eat as many apples as you wish for two or three days. The real detoxification starts after the third day, so see if you can do one more day to benefit from deeper cleansing. You will be surprised to notice that you are not as hungry as you would have expected; this may very well be due to the monotony of the menu! You can still drink your daily amount of water, or two liters or more if you exercise. Herbal teas (only) can be taken as desired throughout the day.

Tip: If you feel blocked up and need to kick-start your bowel elimination, see page 69.

JUICE FASTING is probably the better-known way to detoxify the body. It is pleasant enough; just make sure that you don't use commercial juices, which often have added ingredients, and definitely stay away from concentrates, as moldy fruits are thrown in with fresh ones in the manufacturing process. If you want to do this fast, you need to buy a juicer and make your own fresh juices. This is a valuable investment that will give you regular health dividends!

You can use either fruits or vegetables to make juices; although for digestive purposes, it is better to keep fruits and vegetables separate while you fast. The simpler the food is, the easier it is to digest. In general, fruits are cleansing and vegetables are strengthening for your system. You can vary the kind of fresh produce you use from day to day if you feel that you are getting bored. Try to buy organic, especially while you fast.

Tip: You might develop a taste for homemade juices after this fast, unless you already have! *This us a great habit and a wonderful boost for your health and beauty capital.* A glass of vegetable juice before a meal is very alkalinizing, especially if you are about to have animal protein; it will help to avert an "acid stomach" if you are prone to this.

See *Juicing for Health, The Juicing Detox Diet* by Caroline Wheater (33).

THE MASTER CLEANSE is both the title of a book by Stanley Burroughs (8) and the name of the fast he proposes. It is a longer fast; it needs to be undertaken for a minimum of ten days for best results. Perhaps you should wait until you are familiar with fasting before trying this particular one. It is based on a precise recipe, which includes a mixture of lime or lemon juice, *genuine* maple syrup, cayenne pepper, and water. It is pleasant enough and won't leave you feeling hungry, as it is quite a filling drink. Your energy level will remain quite stable throughout the day, as any drink other than water is basically liquid food, in a readily absorbable form.

Tip: This is quite a practical fast, as you can prepare enough mixture for the day if you are going somewhere or if you are working (just don't bother telling anyone at the office!). It doesn't need to stay in the fridge, as it will not spoil if used within the day. It is not suitable for people with citrus intolerance.

SEVERAL OTHER METHODS OF FASTING are available, such as the Grape Cure. See *The Detox Bible,* an eBook by Chet Day, available at www.chetday.com. This eBook is a journal written by the author while on his fast, which may be handy if you want to give yourself a detailed idea of what to expect, especially if you are new to fasting and on your own.

WATER FASTING is a very efficient method of detoxifying the body, and is known to be the hardest of them all. You will come across huge controversy if you do some research on the subject, but I, among thousands of other people, have done it many times and have had fantastic results. The fear surrounding water fasting is based on a fear of dying shared by a lot of people. But rest assured that no such thing will happen, especially if you are present and therefore in touch with your own body. I love it because a week of this fast (in detoxifying benefit) is the equivalent of double the amount of time doing a juice fast. Water fasting is in fact the only real fast, technically speaking, as there is no liquid food (like fruit or vegetable juice) ingested at all. Personally, I find it easier, as there is no food entering the body at all; once the mind is given a clear message, the action (or non-action) is effortless.

Tip: I find that keeping in contact with food is important while I fast, although some people prefer not to even look at it, which can present a serious challenge, as food is everywhere. You'll be surprised to realize that you have the strength to cook for the rest of the family and, in fact, this could prove to be a valuable distraction to an otherwise long-foodless day. The tactile and olfactory contact with food may fill you up while you fast, because food is such an important daily ritual that it can be quite nice to still have access to it, even if you won't be eating it yourself! You can rest knowing that at some point, you will eat again, with a level of gratitude that you may not have experienced previously.

BREAKING YOUR FAST

There is a definite method to breaking a fast, to make sure that your digestive system can *ease itself* back to regular eating habits. This very much depends on what kind fasting you have completed. For now, we'll assume that you have achieved a one-week water fast. You have just put so much energy into cleansing yourself; it would be a shame to not take adequate care now!

BREAKING A WATER FAST

Part one: Orange juice is the best liquid food with which to break your fast. Again, stay away from concentrates and commercial juices. A few organic oranges squeezed into a glass will do wonders. You won't believe how good something so simple can taste when you haven't eaten for a while … party time for your taste buds! It makes you grateful for the simpler things in life.

Tip: If you are citrus-intolerant, choose another juice that appeals to you. Just make sure it is freshly made.

Part two: As you begin to feel hungry again (when your digestive juices are starting to flow), you can drink more fresh orange juice several times that day. Don't forget to drink your water all the same. Start including some fruits later on that afternoon, one type at a time for easier digestion. You can prepare a vegetable soup and drink the broth by evening of the same day if you really want to eat.

Part three: Start the next day with juices and fruits. You can eat vegetable soup later on, and if you feel up to it, start reintroducing regular food in your evening meal. Stay away from heavy proteins and greasy food, so you don't start loading your system heavily straight away.

Tip: Choosing to keep healthy eating habits after a fast is much easier. You have just cleared the ground for new, healthier habits, which will promote well-being and smooth and glowing skin, and will maintain the appearance of youth while fueling you with renewed energy. Some amount of raw food would be a fantastic bonus if included in your diet on a daily basis. If you eat five or six fruits and vegetables a day, make sure three or more are raw.

BREAKING A FRUIT OR VEGETABLE JUICE FAST

This is slightly different, as you have been ingesting liquid food.

- Start including some salad and/or fruits at lunchtime; then include some cooked food by evening or the next day. Keep the food that you are eating light because you will feel quite sick otherwise.
- The best thing to do is wait a couple of hours to see how your metabolism is processing the food you have just eaten. Bear in mind that the body has had very little digesting to do lately, so be gentle with what you send into your stomach.
- If you feel good, then go ahead and make your next meal almost regular (healthy-regular, that is).

Tip: If you feel bloated, too full, or cramping, adjust the amount and the quality of what you are eating accordingly. Definitely do not go for fried chicken and a glass of beer straight away. It would be a shame and *you will regret it*!

When can you expect regular bowel activity?

Movements should resume within one or two days, as waste needs to build up again in the colon, which is completely empty, especially after a long fast.

Tip: You can always massage the abdomen as shown on pages 70-71 if you feel that elimination is too slow. Don't worry about constipation at this stage.

Subtle benefits acquired as a result of fasting

Fasting is constructive on many levels. By the time you have completed the cleansing ritual of your choice, not only will you feel all the obvious physical benefits, but you will also feel a *firming-up of your willpower*. This experience was really quite an accomplishment and *you did it*! Seeing and feeling the direct and immediate impact that fasting has on your mental, emotional, and physical body is *very empowering*:

- You know how much it took for you to fast, so you will definitely think twice about throwing rubbish into your system.
- You now have the knowledge on cleansing yourself whenever you feel that you have overindulged for a prolonged period of time, such as at Christmas or other festive periods. *The knowledge is with you and you can help yourself, as the power is within your reach.*
- You now know exactly how good you can feel when you take really great care of your body (and it shows!), so the choice is yours as to how you want to live your life. *Your choices are your responsibility and yours only.*
- You now feel that you have enough willpower to do *anything else* in your life that had seemed too challenging prior to your fast. *The reward of building up your willpower is a stronger willpower*!
- You feel an upsurge of inner strength as you realize that you can be self-sufficient in resolving some personal issues. Read the recommended books if you are interested in fasting for serious physical ailments and find a professional practitioner who will assist you.
- You now know have a way to extend your natural life expectancy and its quality.

- You feel grateful to have one of the simplest and most powerful methods for *complete self-rejuvenation* at your own disposal … and it's free!

LIVER DETOX

The "Liver Detox" by Hulda Regehr Clark, Ph.D., is in a category of its own, as it actually cleanses the liver and helps you to expel gallbladder stones naturally, *without surgery*. This is an incredible experience! According to Chinese and Ayurvedic medicine, the liver is where emotions such as stress and anger are processed, so it becomes quite full regularly, even if you eat perfectly well and do not drink or smoke. This is a fantastic treat to give your body twice a year; although it would be great if you managed to do it even once. The best time to do it is in early spring, in the summer, or in the early autumn. Keep a full weekend free for this cleaning ritual because it can be quite strong, especially the first time you do it.

Tip: You can download the exact cleansing instructions from Hulda Regehr Clark free of charge by typing *"Dr. Hulda liver & gallbladder cleanse recipe."* I highly recommend it!

Note: It is very possible that anger (old or new) surfaces while doing this cleansing ritual; this is a fantastic opportunity to free yourself from self-imposed limitations. Use the Emotional Cleansing exercise on page 159.

TOPICS EXPLORED IN SECTION 6

- Detoxifying methods for complete rejuvenation
- Cleansing herbs and foods for an inner spring cleaning
- Fruit and vegetable juice recipe
- Detoxifying baths
- Emotional cleanse
- Liver detox

NOTES

7. A Word on the Enemies of Your Progress: Vampires, Thieves, and Tobacco

BEWARE OF VAMPIRES!

I am not talking about the blood-sucking kind here

But rather the type that draws your energy out until there is no more. They can be people you know: acquaintances, friends, coworkers, and even family in some cases. They are those people who regularly unload their problems on you, mistaking you for their therapist or dumping ground. While sharing some burden with friends is fine, dumping is not. By the time they are finished, they feel better having "unloaded," and you feel drawn out and exhausted. If you are exposed to this kind of treatment on a regular basis, you will look and feel older than your years.

There are several possible causes for this:

- They might not be aware of how needy or draining they really are and may have no boundaries.
- They might be aware of their taxing needy-ness but also know that you are always available to accept the overload.
- They might not know how *not to be* so cumbersome. Their problems are very real for them, and they may need help beyond what you can offer.
- You might feel that they drain you but *you* actually do or say nothing about it—so it would be a good idea to check your own boundaries.
- You might not be aware of what is going on exactly, but simply feel *drained* after spending time with them.
- You might be one of those *people pleasers* who cannot say no. Observe your own participation in this.

Your responsibility in the matter:

- Take responsibility by seeing *how* you feed into the issue.
- See if you can develop some boundaries for yourself.
- If this takes place at work, keep the exchange to a minimum and only relative to necessary topics.
- It is okay to say no.
- Remember you are the only person you have direct control over, so it's up to you to do something about this situation.
- Communication is the best way to let someone know how you feel; just make sure you stay away from accusations and simply state your boundaries or position in the matter.

Tip: Stay alert and grounded while you listen to what is going on; see how it affects your energy. If you feel overwhelmed and out of your depth with what you are hearing, diplomatically suggest an avenue that might benefit the person if you can; or at least let them know that you do not have the capacity to provide adequate assistance. Your honesty may in fact contribute to that person finding the help he or she really needs.

What if the source of stress and drain is at work and/or at home?

It can be particularly taxing if you are regularly exposed to this kind of situation, in which case it might take substantial effort to change things for the better. It can be a big challenge if it means reconsidering your choice of career, your place of work, or a relationship or marriage that is not going anywhere. These are serious issues that may require professional assistance. The first step is, as always, to acknowledge that something does not feel right for you. It is important that *you* do something about it, as *you* are ultimately the only person responsible for *your own well-being and happiness.* You deserve to live in a state of joy and peace. Do not settle for anything less than what you deserve. Do not rely on other people or situations to change in order for you to become happier; it does not work that way.

Communication is essential

Whatever the situation, you need to identify your needs. It is absolutely okay to have needs and more than okay to make sure that your needs are met. While we women walk toward a more independent existence, it seems that we find it increasingly difficult to admit to having needs, and to communicate them. This is something to observe in your own life. Asking for a break, a hand, some time off, or anything else you need is a sign of strength and not weakness, as you might think. Do yourself a favor and give to others *only* when you are filled with energy and naturally overflowing with disposable amounts. If you need to make an appointment with yourself in order to get a few hours of rest and leisure, do it! Ask for help if you have children. Check to see what you are deficient in; is it enthusiasm, joy, laughter, family time, space, contact with yourself?

Once you are in contact with what your needs are:

- Express yourself clearly and kindly: always stay clear of accusing the other party (see the communication section on page 193).
- Ask for your boundaries to be respected; things are not going to change unless you ask.

What if communication does not work?

- There is no point in complaining constantly about something and doing absolutely nothing about it. That drains your energy by 100 percent! If you are not being heard when you express your needs, it is time to take action. Become present and trust that you will know what to do.
- If you have done your very best in communicating and still feel disrespected, unheard, not appreciated, or invisible, it might be a wise to get some help. For example, in the case of a relationship, a counselor might prove valuable if both parties are in agreement.
- If you have done everything in your power and have either

been turned down when you suggested seeking help or got some help but it didn't have the necessary impact, consider giving your energy to someone who appreciates it or to something worth your while.

THIEVES

Dream and ambition thieves

Once again, they are probably people you deal with quite frequently, possibly friends and even family. Most of the time, they operate unconsciously; they tend to knock your efforts and laugh at your dreams because they don't believe you can do it—and somehow you take this on board and your ambition is dampened. Their deeper, more unconscious motive for emitting negative remarks may be that you are trying to succeed where they have failed. A "friend," or a family member who seemed to be there for you when times were hard, resents your achievements and your growing prosperity. That doesn't mean that this person has suddenly turned "bad"; he or she may only be able to operate on *poverty frequency*, unable to accept the blessings that life has to offer, such as joy, money, love, etc. That same person may, in fact, secretly wish to achieve more, but is so identified with deeply ingrained negative beliefs that he or she simply cannot give himself or herself permission to do so and therefore resents people who can—whether this is conscious or unconscious or both.

Some simple suggestions that may work for you:

- You might discuss the issue with the concerned person if you both value the bond between you.
- If you don't think this is possible, keep your plans to yourself, especially if your self-esteem is fragile or recently acquired.
- See it as an opportunity to prove that person wrong by turning perceived adversity to your advantage.

- Love that person from a distance as a last resort!

In general, it is best to be selective about your entourage; life is too short! Surround yourself with people who encourage your dreams and successes. When you spend time with people who are in tune with the flow of life, you feel energized and they do too. Ideas and creation circulate among open-minded and positive people, and good things happen. You deserve nothing less than that.

THE CURSE OF TOBACCO

A considerable tax on your health and beauty capital

You already know of the devastating effects that smoking has on your health. If you are still smoking now, this knowledge clearly did not make an impact big enough for you to stop. So I am not going to enumerate all the possible diseases that you can get due to smoking but simply appeal to your vanity. You picked up this book because you have some kind of interest in your appearance and therefore in your health? Well, let me tell you that there is no cosmetic product that can counteract the effects of tobacco. No amount of surgery, even if you have access to large amounts of money, will get rid of that dried up and leathery effect that too much smoking has on your skin. The number one thing you can do to keep your youthful good looks is to stop smoking. It is free (in fact you will save money) and is one of the secrets to conserving beautiful skin and a vibrant body!

Expect fast results!

You'll be surprised how quickly your skin improves once you stop smoking. This will be an incentive to stay off tobacco, with the added bonus of feeling so much better all around—it would be a shame not to try! It seems to be easier for heavier smokers to stop, probably because they see and feel the benefits quicker. If you are a social smoker and have only two or three a day, you have probably heard everyone around you say, "Hey, don't worry, three cigarettes a day won't kill you! Why should you stop if you enjoy smoking so little?" I used to be a social smoker and found that it took me years to get off those three cigarettes, precisely because of *that kind of remark,* which is completely unhelpful.

Beware and be aware

When you make excuses to defend your habit, just know that it is the *tobacco speaking* through you. If people "kindly"' advise you that you should stay on them because you only smoke the odd cigarette and that it couldn't possibly do you any harm, they are seriously mistaken.

Let's get real!

Smoking is deadly, and it makes you look dreadful. It does not matter what anybody says or thinks to the contrary, they are talking through their addiction. When you have a good meal, or a nice glass of wine, or a piece of your favorite dessert, you get a sense of satisfaction. After smoking a cigarette, if you become alert and feel what your body says to you, you will find that *satisfaction* does not describe the sensation left in you. If you can probe deep enough to detect what is going on after a smoke, you will find that a more accurate description is *relief,* the relief of not feeling the tobacco craving any more. People who are conscious enough to be honest with themselves admit feeling dreadful after a cigarette and nearly always regret it. A monotonous and recurrent self-talk amongst smokers is "I must quit soon."

There are no magic-wands-to-stop-smoking on sale anywhere on the planet

So it is up to you to take responsibility for your own health. There are various techniques that seem to work for different people: hypnosis, patches, etc. Another approach however, which can enable you to rely entirely on yourself, is to become and remain totally conscious while you smoke. I used to smoke and this is what I practiced, so it might help you too.

Smoking meditation

- Stay *absolutely present* while you pull a cigarette out of its packet. Notice your breathing. Observe your own gestures.
- If you roll your own tobacco into cigarettes, smoking requires more concentration as you roll up. This is even better: stay present, make a ritual of it.
- Look at the cigarette for a few seconds before you light up.
- Feel how small and how light it is ... a little paper, and some tobacco.
- Realize the power that it has over you.
- Light it; feel that first drag spread to your lungs, and into your whole body.
- Stay alert as you keep smoking.
- Feel the effects it has on your physical body, listen-in: is your heartbeat changing, do you notice your hands and feet getting cold?
- Observe your energy level and your mood: are they being altered?

If you become profoundly alert each time you smoke, you might start to realize what is happening to you on a deeper, cellular level. In fact you won't have to "give up"; it is more like the addiction *will give you up* because it has no tug on you.

Facts about smoking:

- When you buy and smoke cigarettes or tobacco, you are being robbed of your money, your energy, your health, and your beauty.
- Somewhere, deep down inside, you remember being full

of energy, full of wonder, and ready to bite into each new day. Could it be that you are afraid of your own potential without the tobacco?

- Do not delay in helping yourself because you think that you cannot stop on your own: YOU CAN. Simply remember to stay present.
- You might need to get some support, which is absolutely fine. The first step is to make that decision; it is 90 percent decision and 10 percent action.
- See the Rejuvenating Mind section on page 211.

Tip: Read any of the Allen Carr books on the "Easy Way to Stop Smoking" if you are considering helping yourself. They are all excellent; some are especially designed for men, women, and even teenagers.

TOPICS EXPLORED IN SECTION 7

- Energy vampires and ambition thieves
- Smoking: The biggest tax on your health and beauty capital
- Smoking meditation

NOTES

Chapter Three

ULTIMATE REJUVENATING SECRETS

1. The Beauty of Self-Awareness

Self-awareness is the basis of any productive and peaceful living, which is why it is the underlying current of this whole book. Awareness is the foundation of all other changes, so this is a great tool to *plow your own field* and prepare the ground for all other positive transformations in your life. There is nothing more important than to know that you are *here and now,* as peace and well-being look good on everyone!

Here is a simple exercise to practice as often as you can: let your life become a walking meditation.

The Silent Witness exercise

The simpler the exercise, the more likely you are to remember it. Don't make elaborate plans you cannot keep, so that excuses can come in the way of your practice. There are many times and places you can use to become conscious throughout each day. Literally anywhere, anytime, and any situation will do—the simpler and most repetitive, the better. For example, if you start to associate the phone ringing with remembering to become conscious, you will find that consciousness happens automatically whenever this situation occurs. Here are some examples of simple "life-happenings" that you can turn into your spiritual practice.

Waiting is a great one because waiting engenders feelings of impatience for most of us. So it is a fantastic opportunity to "check in"' and just BE. Being aware of just *being* is effortless. We all *wait* for one thing or another many times a day, every day: at the supermarket checkout, for the computer to load up, for transportation, for a friend, for a phone call, for a result, to cross the road, etc.

Going from one place to another is another regular occurrence for us all every day. Check within to see if you are *united* or completely *split*; are your *thoughts* already *where you are going,* or still *where you came from*? Bring yourself "together" by becoming conscious this instant.

Television watching is a numbing experience on all levels, unless you are watching something that sparks interesting conversation (particularly useful with teenagers) or that teaches you something you can actually use: *Oprah Winfrey* was a great example which I enjoyed watching for many years. In any case, using the mute button every time the ads come on (which is very often), take the opportunity to become present by taking a few conscious breaths. Teach your children to use the mute button and explain that this helps them to not get "programmed" by everything they see. You don't need to go into a talk about becoming alert; they *learn by example,* so just take care of yourself. They are probably more present than you, anyway!

Feeling some seemingly insurmountable feeling. You may have just heard some difficult news; tune into your inner body and keep breathing for a few minutes. *Allow* whatever you are feeling right now; *notice* any inner resistance. This may avert your grasping for your usual pain-numbing device: cigarettes, drink, drugs, food, etc. *Right action always comes out of presence,* so trust that once you have become present, *you will know exactly what to do next*. When you become present, you let *that* which you come from (Divine Intelligence, Source, or God) take over, and the right action can unfold as you stay out of your own way.

There are literally hundreds of different things you do every day that can all be turned into opportunities to become present. All you need to do is to become aware as often as you can. For people practicing this for a number of years, you know that it is very hard to stay aware for long periods of time, so don't worry: the conscious effort of bringing yourself back to being aware is more important than desperately trying to stay aware for long periods of time.

Note: *A Call to Love* by Antony De Mello (24) is filled with simple but powerful self-reflecting meditations.

Eckhart Tolle's book, *A New Earth* (31), is a great self-reflecting tool, as is one of his earlier books, *The Power of Now* (32).

Simple practices to access the present moment

- "Listen in" to your inner body, your heart beating, etc.
- Enter a space of peace and awareness by following your breath.
- Observe yourself: your reactions, your movements, your emotions and thoughts, how you listen to others, etc.

For a few brief seconds, there are no thoughts, no opinions, and no judgment: I compare this to being on a truly relaxing mini holiday. This practice does far more to counteract stress than going to a beautiful location for a holiday with a mind full of negativity and worries.

If you are new to this, be patient with yourself; your rational *thought process* will scream and demand explanations on the purpose of such a seemingly useless exercise. There is nothing you could say to your rational mind that would satisfy it; so don't even try. Simply *live and feel the experience*; little by little, you will experience changes in your life.

Self-Love or the Art of Acceptance

We see beauty with our mind; it is interpreted by our eyes

after it has been filtered through our personal beliefs and values, so this is extremely subjective. We all know that famous expression, "Beauty is in the eye of the beholder"; indeed, this is a very valid statement. It describes to perfection the fascination that people who love each other share for one another: the alchemical magic that makes up the sacredness of couples, which is usually hidden from all onlookers. We will explore the fascinating topic of romantic love shortly, but for now, I want to invite you to use this famous expression on yourself. When you see someone who feels truly at peace with himself or herself, living a fulfilling life, you are observing a similar alchemy: he or she has self-love, or a close relationship with self. He or she is *united within*, at one with himself or herself, at one with the Source or Divine Intelligence. His or her magnetic attraction is powerful, he or she naturally attracts people and situations that allow him or her to explore his or her personal potential in its depth and experience natural abundance on all levels.

Self-love, or the art of acceptance, is a natural extension to being conscious and in a relationship with your Self. It is the central pillar of peace and health, and it is the nourishing root of all other relationships in your life. The quality of love that you share with your partner, family, and friends depends 100 percent on how you feel about yourself. So let us explore this further.

Are you single?

Great! That is a fantastic starting point, which is where it all comes from, from harmonious relationships to disastrous and dysfunctional dramas. I am talking about living and being alone, which is the description of your status—not being lonely, which is an emotional issue. The root of all joy and sorrow is ultimately found in the relationship you have with yourself. Getting to the place where you feel *acceptance* and *unconditional love for yourself* comes from being present in your own life, and is in fact the most important work you can ever do for yourself and others. For many people, self-love is more challenging than feeling love for anyone else. However, this is primordial, for how can you truly share something you don't feel yourself? And how do you hope to have someone feel for you what you cannot feel for yourself? Those are the "hidden cracks" that become more apparent as relationships with partners mature.

The Anatomy of Self

Your energy field is made up of your own personal vibrations; those vibrations come from *your feelings and emotions,* which originate from *your* beliefs, usually rooted in *past experiences.* Most beliefs are limited, as they are based in fearful values absorbed along the way during childhood and in past relationships with others. This acknowledgment constitutes the first step toward change and freedom from personal limitations. The second step is the realization that there is no relationship or love affair more important or defining in your life than the one with self. You attract with your energy field the events and the people that come into your life, so in this light, it is easy to appreciate what kind of vibrations you put out, as it is so perfectly mirrored by what comes into your life. Instead of getting upset and blaming people and circumstances, taking responsibility becomes a priority, and *becoming whole* a vital assignment. Are you not always there when drama shows up in your life?

If you feel resistance while reading these words, think of this: love is not born inside you; it is the current of energy that passes through you, it is *that* which keeps your heart beating. Love is ultimately who you truly are, the only "things" in the way are mental and emotional beliefs, negative projections, or resistance to the natural and undeniable flow of Life. Whether you notice it or not, your inner self is always there, moment by moment, waiting to be loved. Here is a simple and powerful exercise you can practice anytime.

The Inner-Lover Mirror exercise

Find a half hour to do this self-inquiry exercise. If you don't think that you have any available time for yourself, make some: book an appointment with yourself in your diary!

Take a pad of paper and a pen.

Find a pleasant place to sit down, facing a mirror.

If you want to start practicing this without a mirror, you could sit outside in nature or literally anywhere.

Make sure all phones are switched off.

Sit comfortably straight, before the mirror if you choose that option.

When you feel ready, close your eyes, and drop your awareness right into your body.

- Simply notice the flow of air coming in and out of your lungs. Do not try to change or force anything, just be a witness to your breathing rhythm.
- Be aware of your physical contact with the chair (or floor); your feet or legs are resting on the ground.
- Notice how you occupy the space around you—again, *simply observe,* be the *silent witness* and stay away from opinions and judgment.
- When you feel ready, open your eyes and meet your reflection.
- Look at yourself. Notice any resistance, if any. If you keep looking intently, you will bypass the physical and fall straight into the soul.
- Make physical contact with yourself by putting your left hand on your heart and your right hand on your belly. If you are more comfortable swapping hands, then do that.

Ask yourself the following:

- What is there not to love about me?
- Would I like to go on a date with myself?

- Do I have an intimate relationship with myself?

See what you have to say to yourself. Those are huge questions. Have the courage to be totally honest; no one is there to judge you. Refrain from censoring what comes out. If the answer is no to one or more questions, ask yourself what it would take for you to feel differently about yourself. You can write down what comes up for you. Take some time to remain still and let your inner guidance reveal those hidden beliefs. This exercise gives you a very good idea of what needs to be acknowledged in you, and what your self-limiting beliefs are. Look within to feel whether those beliefs empower you, or restrict your potential? This self-revealing exercise is equally useful whether you are on your own or in a relationship. Ultimately, know that *you are the only person you can change* and *are able to transform*. Everything shifts and evolves as your perception widens.

There are many wonderful and diverse roads you can follow on your journey to self-awakening. You have probably tried many. We are all individuals, and what works for one person doesn't for another. No one knows better than you what direction to take next; the only real work you ever need to do at any given time is to become present so you can actually hear your own inner guidance. When there is space inside you, you can feel inner peace; when there is inner peace, there is room for fresh ideas and new visions to come into your life.

No artist can paint on a busy canvas, not even the Divine!

Have trust in your own guidance so you can recognize the next step when it comes? You will be amazed at how easy it is for the right tools to show up in your life. This may take the form of a workshop, some healing, a book, a holiday, a change of job or residence, a flash of inspiration, or whatever else you might need that would benefit you the most. Open the window and see what the wind blows in.

Tip: You need to make some time for your spiritual and emotional self *every day.* This is just as important as any other daily ritual you perform to take care of your physical self, like eating, washing, brushing your teeth, etc. It is often neglected, and this is why you feel "fragmented" or out of touch with yourself. This is more necessary than you can imagine; once you start to take care of yourself in this way, you will feel the importance and the relevance of it. Giving yourself time and love regenerates your spirit, allows you to *feel whole* again, and lights up your inner fire; it leaves you ready to do everything else you have to do more efficiently!

Being alone does not mean you have to be lonely

Loneliness can be described as the *inner resistance* to being alone. Being alone, if you are, is simply a physical description of your life at present, something which can change at any minute. The mental refusal to surrender to this simple fact creates the emotional desperation we call loneliness; and any interaction originating from such a place is tainted with neediness, which is a powerful repellent for any kind of fulfilling relationship.

If you are alone and feeling lonely: start by practicing saying an inner *yes* to your present situation. Do the same if you have a partner and feel alone; you will feel better quickly. Acceptance, releasing, letting-go, making peace, or surrendering are all good words to describe coming to terms with what you are experiencing right now, if it is unsatisfactory. An awareness of your deeper feelings in this moment has brought you the opportunity to notice how removed you are from your true Self. A sense of gratitude can now replace feelings of denial and resistance. It does not mean that things will not change; it simply means that the inner resistance that causes you to experience unhappy feelings or stress is gone. Keep practicing an *inner yes* whenever you feel a restriction within yourself. *Right action* is effortless once you are present and alert. When you connect with the vastness of what you truly are, deep contentment arises within you. You begin to experience your life in the way that is meant for you, whether it is shared or not, which is wonderfully liberating. Fresh solutions and new opportunities (that were probably always there) are more apparent to you when you are more present; you start to contribute to your own well-being. As you keep getting closer to your *inner lover* by deepening your relationship with self, your potential increases and you begin to notice the long-awaited changes. See The Is-ness exercise on page 143.

The dream of unconditional love

For now, and for most people, the belief of unconditional love has not translated into reality; it remains a nice concept at most. There is tremendous confusion when we speak of unconditional love. Some people conveniently misunderstand that it is a free-for-all when it comes to sexual partners (which Tantric sexuality, discussed below, can often be mistaken for), or a flaky means to justify a total lack of responsibility for others. The media today is full of reality TV programs about people at war with their responsibilities—this is a perfect reflection of the deep state of confusion prevalent in so many of us at this time in our evolution. Conditional love is what most people feel and express for each other, meaning that the *degree* of their love depends on the behavior of their partner.

Unconditional love is very different from what most us have experienced, in our upbringing or from other relationships. Simply put, it is to love the person for who they are, and not for the things they do or do not do. This is important to remember, particularly when raising children. This kind of love flourishes in the context of mutual respect, honesty, and enough awareness to recognize one's ego and personal limitations when they come up. Yes, it can be hard work, but it truly is the most rewarding work you can do, again starting with self first. An ability to communicate is essential; and it can be a learned skill if it does not come naturally. True communication is absolutely necessary for any type of relationship to work and to blossom into a more harmonious partnership. Demands and accusations are not placed on each other at the expense of the other's happiness. All parties involved have room and freedom to *grow into more of themselves* in the intimacy of a loving environment, where they are heard, accepted, valued, and respected.

Are we still on track for rejuvenating secrets?

Absolutely—more than ever, in fact! Today, scientific research is advancing fast to prove that our environment, thoughts, and feelings are in fact what dictates our health and, ultimately, the life we live. A positive outlook on life, good health, and radiance have direct roots in your emotional state. You can see this so clearly when someone carries pain and worry on his or her face and in his or her body; inner turmoil is one of the *fastest aging factors* there are. Self-rejuvenation or physical regeneration are most definitely linked to self-awareness, as *peace looks beautiful on everyone* and is, in fact, the central pillar to right living. This is attainable, whether you are on your own or in a couple. We have just seen that awareness and peace, like love, is your natural state. If you do not feel it right now, it is only because there are obstructions or old beliefs in the way, but it is *already there*, within you, *waiting to be acknowledged*.

This whole book is dedicated to YOU, and when I say "*real success unfolds from within,*" the kind of success I am talking about is peaceful living and the expansion of your potential on all levels. Once you are aware and into a close relationship with your Self, your life naturally changes and you can begin to live in the way that was intended for you: tapping into your innermost potential and experiencing right living, right relationships, right income, and radiant health.—in short, the natural abundance that is available to all who are open to it.

TOPICS EXPLORED IN SECTION 1

- The beauty of self-awareness
- The Silent Witness exercise
- Simple practices to access the present moment
- Self-love or the art of acceptance
- The Inner-Lover Mirror exercise

NOTES

2. Conscious Loving

Before we look at the truly rejuvenating aspects of enlightened love and sacred sexuality, let us look at *conscious loving* and acknowledge the challenges that we are facing when it comes to sharing ourselves with another. Many of you know that that the old relationship format has run its course, so let us look at tools you can use to prepare the ground for a new love paradigm.

Love is like an altered state

On a purely scientific level, research shows that the "high" we feel when we are in love is due to a biochemical response in our bodies. We produce more endorphins (chemicals in the brain that make us feel in that super-good mood, where pain seems to be a thing of the past!) and our immune system is said to become stronger because our white blood cells perform better. No wonder we all love to love!

After such excitement, when the initial period of infatuation wears off, a daily relationship can become quite a challenge to sustain. An important fact to understand is that the "happily ever after" does not come automatically and in fact requires diligent work and serious commitment. None of us were born with a manual on "how to handle ourselves in relationships," so it is always a learned experience that some of us are good at, and others less so.

What are the odds of creating the life and the union you are dreaming of while thinking and behaving in your habitual manner?

They are pretty much nonexistent. One aspect of insanity, as is famously known by now, is to try to find solutions with the same mindset that created the issue… a common occurrence among people we call "sane"! You are conditioned by your system of beliefs, your values, your past, and your expectations… try living a peaceful life and having loving relationships with all that! The understanding most of us have about love and true connectedness is still extremely limited. Old patterns and expectations tend to creep in unannounced, as discussed in the previous section, even with relatively aware partners and the best of intentions. For many, eventually with time, one or both partners give up and another separation occurs. Or else people stay together, bound by the invisible ties of codependency, and spend most of their time miserable inside, wishing themselves out of the present moment and situation—a sad and difficult life for all involved.

A select few manage to share a fulfilling and joyful life, which is a wonderful thing. They would all admit that it took a substantial amount of conscious efforts to give harmony a chance to rise and develop. A harmonious relationship is possible when both partners have a real but often learned ability to communicate their feelings and ideas without accusations or judgment. Keeping or cultivating an open mind can increase the potential for mutual trust, which can in turn open the space for a deeper, more loving and intimate relationship. *An open mind reflects an open heart*. A commitment to being open and honest in your feelings and an ability to share them with your partner also increases the intimacy potential between you. A reasonable amount of self-awareness enables each partner to stay present in times of conflict and allows emotional maturity to develop, meaning that there is an ability to take responsibility for personal issues. Unfortunately, most people find taking responsibility too much like hard work and would rather substitute it with denial or finding an affair or a new partner. They are traveling through life with a huge "rucksack of unresolved personal stuff," also known as "emotional baggage," ready to unpack at the next stop—a tiring and joyless affair for all involved.

We may have moved a little from the childish and older mind-set concept of "happily ever after" found in all childhood fables and still present in popular romantic fiction, but we have not quite reached a new era when it comes to relationships. We are presently going through an enormous amount of change in the rise of consciousness, and this is very much reflected in the challenges between men and women and in the nature of relationships. The romantic tales portrayed through the medium of storytelling are still reflecting the old mind-set for the most part; a select few address the depth of love and relationships, and none deal with the sacred aspect of sexuality. The main topics covered in stories of the heart usually describe predictable romantic comedies, the platonic or dark side of sexuality, terrible tragedies, or else the traditional epic romance where one or both partners die. Is true love so powerful that death has to take it out of our hands, lest we be unable to survive it?

I don't think so!

Most people ache *to love* and *to be loved*

—Even those of you who are in relationships, so what to do? One of the fast tracks to being happier and having a more fulfilling relationship is to drop expectations around what it *should look like* or what it is *meant to be*. In most relationships expectations are high, giving rise to unrealistic fantasies, while nothing tangible is done to improve or nourish the union at hand. Most people who have true love in their lives report being surprised by the shape it took; it was definitely not *when* or *who* they expected, and all report that it takes a good deal of work and commitment to keep things alive. A relationship needs dedication and positive energy to blossom, just like a green plant needs water to grow; there isn't one organic thing on the planet that survives without nourishment.

Relationships are not a magic wand for "ready-made happiness," as we have been programmed to believe. In fact, expecting happiness through another person is the fastest and surest way to drain yourself, the companionship, and put years on all involved. A relationship is an opportunity for *personal* and *mutual healing*, a ground on which *both partners can grow into more of who they are*, and a doorway into harmony, fun, and freedom. Your partner is ultimately the mirror in which *all you need to become aware of* is reflected back to you, and vice versa. The journey that is made up of your communal life can become an amazing experience once you accept this and begin to witness and consciously participate in the process. A shift in perception can open up access to previously unavailable experiences, and both the relationship and the partners can start to experience deep regeneration and rejuvenation on all levels, for Love is the stuff of Life!

Note: Have a look at my You Tube Channel (MahayanaIDugast) for a short video on Love and Self-Love. Also check Doctor Robin L. Smith's book Lies at the Altar (29), which can be used as a great self-revealing tool.

Working consciously on a relationship

This can be very rewarding, especially where both partners can communicate openly and show respect for one another. Understanding the psychological aspect of love can be very useful, as we all have various baggage from childhood and previous relationships that we haven't always managed to shift. Often, and with the best of intentions, those patterns reemerge after the initial period of bliss is over, which can be anything from a few weeks to several years, depending on the depth of the connection. Being able to understand how to identify the "programming" you carry into relationships is a valuable tool. Once you begin to understand how you function within any particular relationship, your patterns are highlighted and you are able to be present to your own reactions, which is healing in itself. Emotional maturity begins when you take responsibility for your own feelings.

Note: *Getting the Love You Want,* by Harville Hendrix, Ph.D. (17), may literally save your relationship, if read in time. I read it years after being separated, but it was still self-revealing for my own patterns and those of my ex-husband's in the relationship; the reading resulted in freedom in the form of radical forgiveness. I highly recommend it!

The couple as a team

The union talked about here is one that allows you to retain your individuality while merging with the other. Too many relationships fail because one or both partners merge with one another in such a way that they lose a lot of their personal identity, and therefore suffer from self-denial. Each one of us is only too familiar with the expression: "Here is Mary or Jack with her/his other half. " Who really wants to be just a half!? Real union sees the couple as a *team,* each contributing to the other's well-being, progress, and personal success. If the relationship you are in right now takes away from who you truly are, you are compromising yourself. Sharing your life with someone surely must allow you to *flourish and be more of yourself,* and not less. Take a moment to reflect on this and see if you are satisfied with your life.

Passionate partnership

To achieve any kind of harmony, both partners need to make a commitment to working at nourishing their union. The reward is a relationship that is enjoyable and far more productive for both parties, naturally providing each person with *tools for growth.* As previously explored, positive communication needs to be exchanged, based on one's feelings rather than an accusative analysis of the other's behavior.

Communication: The fuel of intimacy

Don't expect your partner to be psychic and know how you feel; he or she dealing with his or her own challenges and often does not realize how important an issue may be for you. Do not assume that your partner understands what you are going through just because you have been together for some time; make some space to discuss your needs with each other in a relaxed setting, when both of you have time and are not in a state of severe emotional upheaval. *TALKING is important, LISTENING is vital;* it is better still if both are practiced in a state of presence.

See the Body and Soul Connecting ritual on pages 208-209.

Example: When you need to communicate something you feel to your loved one (children, partner, parents, friend, etc.), make sure that you do not merge the behavior with the person, e.g., "I hate *you* when *you* … " versus "What you said brings up … *in me; I feel* … (hurt, sad, angry, etc.) and what I need from you is …" This can be a challenge to practice, particularly if it is new in your relationship. You may even require the professional assistance of a coach to get you started.

Exercise of appreciation

Before going to sleep at night, tell your partner one, two, or even three things you appreciate about him. He or she may do the same in return. We tend to focus on what is not right in self and others, which only serves to magnify the negative feelings that hold us apart. Instead, focus on what is right or lovable in the other, even if you can only think of a few qualities for now—it's a start! Implementing this positive practice invites mutual feelings of gratitude and appreciation, and helps to cleanse any negativity which might otherwise hold you resentful and unable to sleep peacefully.

If you are not in a relationship, you can do this for yourself. Write down three things that you appreciate about yourself; you'll be surprised at how amazing you really are when you read your own notes a while later. This is also a great practice to use with children, and useful with teenagers in helping them to develop a sense of gratitude. You'll get a few moans and groans, but you might also get a few laughs!

Note: I love Gay and Kathlyn Hendricks' fun and powerfully transformative practices for couples. Have a look at www.hendricks.com for short videos, and other materials you can use.

TOPICS EXPLORED IN SECTION 2

- Conscious loving
- The couple as a team
- Communication: The fuel of intimacy
- Exercise of appreciation

NOTES

3. Sacred sexuality and its regenerative power

Let us look past limited beliefs and explore ourselves deeper…

The Tantric and Taoist traditions offer different ways of accessing personal freedom through the practice of sacred sexuality, which can be healing and regenerating for both partners, individually and mutually. Love is a state that is inherent in us all, and you can begin to enjoy feeling it right now by becoming still, taking a breath, and connecting with your own energy. Do the same when you are in the presence of your partner; you can then feel his or her *deeper being*, which means that a very different kind of union is possible.

See the Body and Soul Connecting ritual on pages 208-209

Love passes through you like an everlasting current of energy; *love and presence are one and the same*. You don't feel it all the time because you are too busy criticizing yourself (and others) or playing out various mental fictional scenarios of yesterday and tomorrow—all of which take you out of the present moment and nearly all of which make you feel ill at ease. Your best ally or "safety rope," as discussed in the introduction of this book, is to simply remember to connect to your inner source. The only real challenge you have is to *remember to do it*! But more and more, as you awaken by becoming conscious, you begin to feel a new kind of vibrancy, a renewal, like a new lease of life. You are far more susceptible to *attracting love* when you can feel it within yourself. You are far more likely to attract someone who has a similar connection to his or her own self, and therefore you will have an opportunity to create the kind of relationship you have been dreaming of.

Sexual energy can be healing and deeply regenerating

It can enhance the quality of your life, be empowering and regenerative, and even extend your current expectation of longevity. I am not talking about the *commercial commodity* that sex has become today, but of something far deeper.

Sexuality is a subject that houses enormous taboos in many cultures. There can be a lot of pain around the sexual act for men and women alike, so understanding this powerful energy is beneficial for all (including teenagers). Let us explore two ancient traditions, the Taoist and Tantric, which both include the act of lovemaking as part of an expansion of consciousness.

TAOISM

Taoist philosophy is believed to be the most ancient system of knowledge on earth and has been practiced for over 6,000 years

Its teachings offer a way to achieve well-being, self-awareness, complete rejuvenation, and mutual healing; and a practice to attain freedom from the mind, also known as enlightenment. The exercises taught in this holistic philosophy focus on the organs, the energetic systems as well as the more subtle auric fields rather than the physical appearance of a person. For indeed, what use is a lovely, toned body if the liver or the heart does not function properly?

Bringing ritual into your daily life

If you are working with the aim of self-awakening, you already know that taking good care of your body comes completely naturally; you wouldn't have it any other way. When you truly understand that your body is the house of your spirit (I call it your body-temple), *your desires get closer to your needs and your potential naturally increases*. You naturally want to live your life with as much awareness as can be practiced. Think of this:

you would not go and pour some tar or empty your weekly rubbish over your beautiful garden or your favorite place of worship, whether it be at home, in church, or in any temple ... so why do it inside your own body?

If you find that you still are prone to acting as your "old self" and are experiencing difficulties moving through some deeply ingrained patterns, remember this: you are no less than a manifestation of the Source, a spark of the Creator. What if the Divine came over for dinner tonight? How would your house look and feel? Just know that you deserve no less.

See the Creating Sacred Space ritual on page 206.

Mainstream sexuality versus conscious sexuality

You may be surprised and delighted to know that *making love consciously* is a vehicle for self-healing and a potent rejuvenating factor. More often than not, sex is used (or misused) as a tool for power/control, to get a "release," or to make up after an argument; none of these purposes serves a truly loving and caring relationship. Most of us were raised with the idea that sex is a means to an end, a vice, or something forbidden that should not be talked about at all. Many religions classify sex as a sin. In a lot of households, where domestic relationships are "relatively okay," sex is often used as a bargaining tool. I say "relatively okay" because the minute that either partner gives or takes sex without awareness, it is devoid of any nurturing qualities and in some cases can be a kind of *conscious rape.* I know that it is a harsh way of putting it, but there will not be any conscious evolution unless we become aware of what needs to change.

Take a moment to scan the "joy level" in and around you before you let your usual defense mechanisms block the way for transformation. There is at present a wind of urgency beckoning you to awaken, so now is the time to become completely honest with how you want your life to play out, and what kind of relationship you want to experience.

Pornography is now available mainstream and is currently being portrayed as a tool to increase sexual arousal for anyone short of inspiration. It has even been renamed "erotica" to make it more marketable, which further contributes to the already enormous pornographic entertainment industry. This is both a worrying and a dramatically negative evolution, which can only lead to further confusion and ultimately more separation, both personal and mutual. Pornography focuses exclusively on the external mechanics of sexuality, momentarily quenching thirsty egotistical minds. In order to feel satisfied, the mind creates scenarios where pain, humiliation, or danger prevail—in short, any challenging situations or sensations that might make one feel more alive—in a desperate attempt to escape the daily numbness of being. The more anaesthetized the body feels, the stronger the stimulus has to be. Sadly, this current state of confusion is a reflection of the deficit that most people feel inside themselves. Unless there is an awakening of consciousness, the contact with the inner self remains lost, leaving too much space for unconsciousness or negative creativity in one's life.

Let us note that *too many children and adults are already the victims of this mind-set,* so how about contributing to the rise of positive sexual awareness through your awakened perceptions? As an individual, you have all the power you need to change this by simply allowing consciousness to shine through you and in your own life: this is the root of all permanent change.

Our energies are interconnected and all events taking place *anywhere* at any given time feed into *collective consciousness: we are all ONE.*

The world needs your contribution.

Sacred sexuality

You may believe in God, you may not; it really does not matter: life force is indisputably in and all around us, and we are definitely alive by some invisible grace. There are many names for God or this invisible energy, since our species is extremely diverse and we therefore perceive things in our own individual ways, which is wonderful. For any of us to manifest into physicality, Natural Intelligence orchestrates an intricate symphony of Creation that can only be described as Divine. Each time any of us has the privilege of witnessing creation, we are in awe.

Divine creation happens when we are *inspired*, connected to the *source*, or in tune with *that* which we came from. This need not apply only to the conception of a child, although it is a very different experience for all concerned if a soul is consciously invited or received. Some of you, conscious parents, have had the privilege of that experience. Creation, once unleashed, may take any form that is accessible to you and in tune with your individual talent. This is when *natural prosperity* can flow into your life. Making love consciously is a most fulfilling experience on all levels, where both partners feel *nourished and empowered.* Lovemaking is the most sacred vehicle of communication between two souls, allowing Divine Energy to fill our beings with its illuminating presence. It is the magical fusion that inspires so many works of art, and that so many people long for: a taste of the journey home.

A little death

In England, during Elizabethan times, making love was called "dying." Elizabethans associated the orgasm that literally sweeps us *out of our mind* with death. This is not a bad analogy, as it is possibly the only time when control is totally relinquished, when the act of letting go is authentic, and we are briefly in a state of complete *being*. Allowing your body to be a conscious vessel of creative energy can be such a powerful experience that it is potentially *life altering*. This applies to you, whether you have a partner or not. Sharing pleasure with a loved one is obviously more fun, but *self-cultivation* (Taoist term for self-pleasuring) is a healthy and natural vehicle to access your creative potential and tap into your own source of joy. *This is one of the best self-rejuvenating secrets!*

Refine your personal mantra

Many of us were raised to believe that suffering is required in order to attain peace and freedom. It is true that you need to become sick of your own sickness to truly awaken, but once you experience alertness and begin to enjoy moments of presence, or thoughtless-awareness, you may refine your personal mantra. You can choose to tune into "joy frequency" and start to learn out of pleasure, fun, and creativity rather than all the negative alternatives you formerly required. This may be an important statement to include in your self-talk or meditative practice. The old love format which is selfish, clingy, ego-ridden, all–consuming, and potentially destructive becomes totally obsolete—for why would you want to burden yourself with anything less than what you deserve?

See the Gratitude Prayer on pages 215-216.

Society according to Taoist philosophy

This tradition offers practical ways to live, starting within each individual, with a view to global wellness (planet rejuvenation!). Simply put, the Taoist view that when there is personal fulfillment, there is peace; where there is peace, there is harmony between people; where there is harmony between people, there are balanced families; balanced families make for a more productive society and ultimately a very different type of nation from what we have been experiencing until now. It makes great sense to put attention and energy in the only place where real change is possible: YOURSELF. The rest will unfold in the light of new awareness; as mentioned previously, trying to change anything external with the same limited amount of consciousness is a sure recipe for failure. Success, on the other hand, arises when you merge with your innermost potential and work in fusion with the Source.

Know thyself!

Within Taoist philosophy, there are many different exercises that both women and men can individually practice to strengthen their sexual organs and remedy some delicate issues. Irregular and abnormally painful menstrual cycles, impotence, or premature ejaculation can all be helped by using simple methods that cost absolutely nothing but a little study and, of course, some practice. They offer a very empowering alternative to pain-killers and various other drugs used to "fix" manifested problems.

Women can start to enjoy the multileveled orgasms they have the capacity to access—a doorway to unlimited pleasure. The result of such communion is sexual ecstasy but also feelings of deep joy, profound mutual nourishment, intimacy, peace, access to co-creative energy, and of course: *indisputable rejuvenation*! For a lot of women, most of the pleasure received while making love originates from attention given to the clitoris, so the good news is that even if you are on your own, you can have plenty of pleasure right now! Every woman has the potential to enter into ecstatic states by giving herself *unlimited pleasure* through self-cultivation. Knowing yourself intimately also gives you more confidence about communicating your preferences when sharing time with a lover. Consider this your homework assignment!

Men can develop the capacity to augment their pleasure and enhance their sexual performance, control their erection and ejaculation for prolonged bliss, and reduce the depletion of energy usually felt after lovemaking. It enhances both partners' ability to access their personal and mutual potential on all levels and in all areas of their lives, from the most mundane and practical to the most refined spiritual realms. The bond made by dedicating all your mutual energies to serve one another builds the foundation for a solid and fulfilling relationship and a happy and healthy family.

This was knowledge that the Yellow Emperor (2697–2598 BC) knew very well how to utilize. It inspired his whole existence and gave him the supreme ability to access his full potential during his lifetime. He lived an inspiring one hundred years and is said to have reached immortality. I hope that this makes you curious to research conscious sexuality. See all recommended books below for a great start. Keep it fun and enjoy!

Note: For further studies on Taoist philosophy and practice, I recommend Dr. T. Chang's book, *The Tao of Sexology, The Book of Infinite Wisdom* (11), which is full of practices and exercises.

See also Mantak Chia's book, *Cultivating Male Sexual Energy* (12), for more inspiring practices.

Fear around sexuality

A lack of confidence in one's own sexuality can bring up fear and be a stumbling block for a lot of people. This could have begun earlier on, during childhood, when parents prevented the toddler from "playing with himself or herself," unable to accept this natural process because of their own beliefs. Fear around sexuality can also be linked with unpleasant memories linked to past trauma, or it can result from a personal or cultural heritage of shame around the body. Patience and perseverance are required to loosen up years of set belief and traumatic memories in some cases. Taoist wisdom is powerful in its simplicity. It offers a clean and natural approach with simple exercises to help you get in touch with yourself.

Fear around sexuality can equally affect people who think themselves as "spiritually evolved." It can show up as a lack of emotional investment in a relationship, or can sometimes manifest as a complete severance from any sexual activity altogether (often for religious purposes). In other cases, the act of love can be performed "relatively well," meaning that it provides some amount of physical pleasure but remains hollow—mechanical and completely lacking in intimacy. And yet, the fear of intimacy, which is generated by various mental and emotional negative beliefs, can be used as the doorway to get into a more fulfilling relationship … the kind of connection that you keep wishing for and that keeps eluding you. Remember this great saying (author unknown): *"**That** which blocks the way **is** the way'."*

Tip: Before engaging in any sexual activity with another person, check that you have the capacity and readiness to open your mind fully to the experience, and that it is indeed what you want at this point. It is high time that lovemaking be recognized as a sacred ritual and be treated with corresponding respect. If you don't feel ready or able to share yourself with another, trust and respect your own feelings, and communicate kindly with your partner.

See "Creating Sacred Space" and the Body and Soul Connecting ritual at the end of this chapter.

TANTRA, THE ART OF CONSCIOUS LOVING

Tantra is an ancient spiritual practice where sexuality is included in rituals to attain self-awareness, self-regeneration, and unity within, and to access freedom from the mind. The Tantric movement originated in Tibet and came down through Hindu and Buddhist traditions. It later spread through China. The fact that sexuality is included in this practice has been confusing for the interpreting Western mind. It is fair to say that whenever scholars study ancient cultures and traditions, they can only interpret the wisdom perceived according to their own level of awareness, which is nearly always limiting, no matter how academically accomplished they may be. While tantra has begun to reemerge into global awareness, it has mainly been associated with "the yoga of sex" and is commonly thought of by most people as "gourmet sex." While there is nothing wrong per se with either of these descriptions, it has to be said that they are both desperately stifling labels, poorly describing such vast wisdom.

Tantra pertains to the *expansion in all things,* with the ultimate goal being balance, unity, and harmony within yourself primordially and subsequently for the rest of your life. Rejuvenation, deep nourishment, liberation are all on the menu for the dedicated student. This spiritual practice is based on the wisdom that we are in a relationship with all things; it reminds us that our own bodies mirror the cosmos, from the macrocosm to the microcosm: "As above, so below."

Practicing Tantra

The allowing of sexuality into one's spiritual practice is not without serious challenges, as passion can give rise to a great many obstacles. This path is an intense one and is definitely not for the faint-hearted. The principal requirement for such a practice is an absolute desire to fully awaken: to lift the veils that cloud clear vision and intuitive living. This process, just like any other self-awakening practice, can manifest itself in the form of very challenging situations, usually accompanied by huge personal resistance until illusionary perception disintegrates to make space for awakened clarity. Patience, perseverance, laughter, and playfulness are all of the essence.

Unlike some spiritual traditions, true Tantric practitioners allow themselves the use of alcohol and animal produce in their rituals: they drink wine, tear through red meat with appetite and passion, dance, and live a life that is both fierce and free from judgment!

Women in Tantric Buddhism

In the true Tantric tradition, and again unlike most other spiritual practices, initiated women are not only respected but are in fact recognized as God in female form and worshipped as such. Such women also know men to be God in male form, and both partners understand that *spiritual liberation is a mutual matter*. The initiator behind each and every self-realized man has always been a woman. This realization (or remembrance) is not to be used for self-enhancement or ego-inflation, lest it would instantaneously block the recipient from any real access to freedom and realization.

Tantric philosophy sees each of us as a spark of Divine Consciousness. This realization in itself can be sufficient to put an end to all pain and patterns incurred by self-doubt, and bring into manifestation the self-esteem that renders looking for outer sources of approval unnecessary. The peace and freedom so ardently pursued in the external world is *experienced within*. By realizing your primary nature, which is that you are pure consciousness encapsulated in bodily form, the kind of trust that emanates from you is one of magnetic quality. This magnetic quality becomes apparent in your daily life when all manifested events and challenges are recognized as your *teachers*—all available to help you liberate yourself through *a reduction of identification with form*. A union built on these foundations houses considerable differences from the traditional and sadly limited views of current companionship. The mutual love and respect born of such union enables both partners to truly experience unconditional love and live a life that is productive, peaceful, and graceful.

Note: If you are interested in this powerful wisdom, read *Passionate Enlightenment* (28) by Miranda Shaw for a truly expansive comprehension of authentic Tantric tradition.

So what about wild sex?

You have probably come across the *Kama Sutra*, which can be imposing, especially when you see postures where people seem to be dismembered! The real practice of *conscious loving*, however, does not focus on sexual techniques. It is simply based on an ability to merge energetically with each other before anything physical happens. Both partners use conscious breathing to stay connected and present with one another. Everything else can be improvised! Fun is just as important as anything else in life, and it is a well-known fact that delicious dishes are created from happy mistakes; the same goes for creative loving. Don't worry about '"getting things right," keep it light hearted—especially if you are trying new approaches with an existing partner.

This is a real treat that will make you look and feel years younger!

While you may not be inclined to delve deep into Tantric tradition, there is certainly much to be gained by reading and practicing a little from its powerful wisdom. The following two rituals are inspired from Tantric wisdom; they are fun and powerful to practice, and they may bring a new dimension to your existing partnership or prepare the ground for one to come into your life if you are on your own at present. Have fun!

Creating Sacred Space

The idea behind creating *sacred space* is to introduce ritual into your love life, to rekindle your mutual passion. I am not suggesting that spontaneity should be discounted; on the contrary, always go with the flow! This is simply about putting some energy back into your partnership, gifting each other with real soul nourishment. Make sure that you have both communicated on this and expressed mutual interest, as surprises are not always appreciated. You need a couple of hours to yourselves, without the children or anyone else calling. Pick a room where you can have full privacy and in which you both feel comfortable. Make sure you turn off all phones.

- Start by bringing your attention to the present moment, focusing your intention on the task at hand. You can use various tools to help you clean the room: purification by smoke from a smudge stick works well (smudge sticks are bundles of dried sage used by Native Americans to purify spaces and people), burning some incense, using bells, or simply beating on a saucepan (which is slightly noisier but just as fun!). Keep doors and windows open so the energy can move out. This is even more important if confrontations have occurred in that room. This cleansing ritual is equally important when staying in a hotel or moving into a new house.

- Use some colorful drapes and plenty of cushions and soft blankets so you can lie down comfortably. You may like to use the floor in front of the fireplace covered with a nice rug.
- Keep some light refreshment nearby for convenience and enjoyment. Bring in a beautiful bowl full of some of your favorite juicy fresh fruits, a jug of water, some honey, a glass of champagne, or a little wine (too much of it will lower your energy), or anything else you might fancy.
- Lighten the place up with soft tones—a silk scarf draped over a lamp can dim bright lights and, of course, candles are always beautiful. Scented candles can add to the atmosphere, if you like them. Make sure they are out of the way for later, when you are in the throes of passion!
- If you want to celebrate in abundance, cover a small area with flower petals of all kinds. Rose petals are rather decadent but impart great sensory delights if you are in an extravagant mood!
- Make a beautiful massage bland using some sweet almond oil mixed with a few natural essential oils of your choice. Sensual oils include rose Otto, neroli, ylang-ylang (very overpowering, so use sparingly), geranium (also strong), sandalwood, jasmine, cardamom, and patchouli. A gorgeous blend can be made using two drops of rose oil, three drops of sandalwood, and one drop of ylang-ylang into a tablespoon of almond oil.

- Have some music ready at hand if you like; select something that you would both find appealing. One of you might play an instrument, in which case you can play a piece of music for your partner.
- Enhance the space with a few feathers and flowers.

You may like to have a bath or shower on your own or together before you meet in this beautiful *sacred space* that you have created. Change into something light and comfortable, made with natural fiber, like silk or cotton, that allows you to move freely. The mood might move you to dance for each other seductively or together … the possibilities are endless! The simple fact that you are uniting your energies to create a space for your mutual enjoyment is beneficial in itself. Be like children; get creative in building your playground and spending time with each other.

Body and Soul Connecting ritual

The aim of this practice is to make yourself *whole* before you proceed with any situation, before love-making, when in a difficult state of mind, before communicating with your partner, or simply to replenish your energy. It can be performed on your own or with a partner.

With a partner

Each of you can do the following while sitting, standing, kneeling, lying down, or however you feel most comfortable:

1. Face your partner.
2. Press the palms of your hands together lightly before your heart.
3. Close your eyes and become present by getting in touch with your breathing.
4. When you feel ready, open your eyes and look into the eyes of your partner.

5. Keep breathing and looking at each other for a few moments.
6. Your breathing may attune with your partner's—a beautiful experience. Don't worry if it does not, though.
7. When you feel ready, bend forward and let your foreheads meet.
8. Extend your hands forward and touch your partner's heart with the tips of your joined hands. He or she makes the same gesture.
9. Feel your energies connecting, your souls merging.
10. Salute each other with your own words or "I salute the Divine in you …".'
11. Move back when you feel ready: you are now in the space of *connected presence.*

In the ancient Mayan language, recognizing the Divine in the other is expressed in this greeting: "In Lakesh," which means "I am another yourself." You can also use "Namaste" from the Hindu tradition or "Aloha" from the Hawaiian tradition, as they have similar meanings. Any of these can be used in step 10.

Without a partner

The same steps apply; you can place yourself before a mirror. For step 8, replace touching your partner's heart with touching the ground before you. Feel the earth-energy nurture your whole being.

Note: Margo Anand has a whole lifetime of experience in Tantric practice. She has made this ancient wisdom beautifully accessible to Westerners through workshops and books. Two of my favorite books are *The Art of Every Day* Ecstasy (2) and *The Art of Sexuality* (3). Check out www.margotanand.com for more information.

TOPICS EXPLORED IN SECTION 3

- Sacred sexuality and its regenerative powers
- Taoism
- Tantra, the art of conscious loving
- Creating Sacred Space exercise
- Body and Soul Connecting ritual

NOTES

4. The Rejuvenating Mind

Our basic functioning mechanism

As spirits having a human experience, we are privileged with a mental, emotional, and physical body.

- The mental body is where all concepts, designs, and beliefs are held in the form of thoughts.
- The emotional body literally "links up" the mental body to the physical body via feelings.
- The physical body is the last to be affected in response to the emotional body.

This is valid for absolutely anything and is fundamentally how we materialize our reality, from an illness to the design and building of a house. The emotional body is very important and is where all connectivity happens; I call it "the glue" because nothing can really come into your life until you feel it first. Of course, all the above are far more powerful if you let in the spiritual element, our Creator; meaning that you "stay out of your own way," particularly when you are in need of healing or regeneration, which this section aims to help you achieve. Being guided by the Creator or Source in yourself feels like inspiration; the word *inspiration* comes from the Latin *spirited,* which means "from spirit." This is more evident when you enjoy great works of art that have been created in this way, such as music, paintings, innovative thoughts, etc.

You + Creator or Source = Success.

Once you are inspired, what you need to do (or not do as the case may be) becomes evident and may take any form that looks like a solution to you.

THE POWER OF CREATIVE POTENTIAL

Goal setting

- Make your decision (make sure you are 100 percent positive).
- Write it down: simplicity and clarity are essential.
- Keep your mind open and alert so you can be receptive to the solution, the support, or the tool when it shows up in your life.
- Relax and trust that it is on the way; thinking about it obsessively always slows down its fruition, and doubting it literally cancels it.
- Get into action when inspired.

Once the decision is made clearly, the support you need appears in your life, effortlessly. You have probably experienced this before: for example, when someone gives you a book on a topic in which you recently developed an interest ... amazing synchronicity, wasn't it?

Asking clearly and precisely for what you need works well, *particularly when it contributes to your well-being and the development of your awareness and potential.* Make absolutely sure that you stay out of your own way (let the Creator in) for it to take effect within yourself and in your life. You might have a couple of lists at home: a monthly and a yearly one. Start with small things. State clearly what you want to achieve and put the list away for some time. Soon enough, when you revisit your list, you will be able to notice changes and evolution in your life, which feels great because it give you more positive beliefs. This is very empowering and has a knock-on effect when you see that it really works; you start to realize that *life is conspiring to bring you all that you need,* once you are clear, conscious, and receptive with an opened mind.

For some of your bigger goals, it is best to leave the list aside and check only on a yearly basis; you'll be surprised and amazed at how much has come true for you. Bigger visions often need time to incubate, so patience and trust are essential ingredients to your success.

Example extracted from my personal list of goals

A few years back, I was already in pretty good form—doing some exercises most days, eating healthily—but I still smoked about three cigarettes a day. My wish was to be 150 percent physically fit, so I wrote this down as one of my goals. I purposely left out *how exactly* I was going to make that happen because had I tried quite a few things that did not work out.

A few months down the line, having quite forgotten about it, I found myself enjoying a brisk walk around the park after I dropped the children into school. When I actually thought about it, I noticed that I was walking forty-five minutes *every day* and no longer felt like smoking every day. I felt so refreshed when I came home that a smoothie seemed far more appealing than a cigarette and another coffee. I did not lay out a drastic new routine for myself (I really don't think that those work for very long anyway), I simply wrote down my decision. It was 90 percent decision, 10 percent action.

Have you been praying or asking without success?

Can you really manifest the reality you want? Yes and no.

Yes, because the ability to see desires manifested in your life is simply based in the allowing of them—meaning knowing how to stay out of your own way, or surrendering.

No, because if things are not happening for you, you are probably asking from *a place of deficit*. If you ask for something that you do not feel, you will not receive it, since, as we have just explored, the emotions are the glue between the mental and physical body.

Gratitude plays a huge part on all levels, so if you are asking for a healing, for example, make sure you start your prayer or meditation with something for which *you feel true gratitude*; and only then proceed to welcoming what you are expecting with as much gratitude.

This is the Master key.

In truth, you are perfect now and so is your life. How can I say that? Because you are who you are and your life is what it is; therefore it is exactly as it is meant to be for now. *Otherwise it wouldn't be*. Remember that saying "no" to *what is* is the main source of stress in your life; reality happens whether you agree with it or not and exists to show you what you have been thinking about and feeling. If you are unhappy with yourself, your life, or both—this is perfect, because you are being pushed to awaken. With great gifts come great responsibilities! Your life, being what it is at this time, is the sum total of the thoughts and emotions you have had until now. But of course this can change as you *intend* on experiencing transformation by starting to work on yourself—the only person you can control in your life. Apparent "problems" manifest in your life as tools and teachers for your own personal growth, and when you can smile at *seemingly negative events* taking place in your life, you are no longer being pushed around by your own mental and emotional conditioning, and you can start to live in peace and natural abundance. Real success unfolds within you. Peace is inherent within you; it is only your mind that says otherwise.

See the "Is-ness" exercise on page 143 and the Gratitude Prayer on pages 215-216.

Needs versus wants

Until you awaken, your desires are rarely in tune with your needs. Most desires or wants are formulated by ideas and concepts that are not even yours; some you might not even like if they were to materialize because you may not be ready or able to sustain them. A great example of that is winning the lotto, or a large sum of money, which is high on so many people's wish list. Because they have no previous experience with handling such large amounts of money, they often lose it all quickly, while incurring extra debts.

The best use of your energy is in removing personal resistances, staying present and connected, and welcoming whatever comes into your life. As you live an aware life, in close relationship with yourself, imbued with inspiration, new abilities, solutions, and real durable change can come into your life, tailor-made to your own ability to receive, utilize and enjoy. If you have got this far in life, and are managing to read this, you have everything you need to prosper. As you keep observing the obstacles imposed by your mind materializing into your physical reality, and realize that they are your teacher and do not define you, a new life begins. Your life transforms effortlessly as your perception widens. You are on the road to success.

Gratitude Prayer

This is a soul rejuvenating prayer. You can read it twice a day, before going to sleep and upon awakening—when your mind is the most receptive, in an alpha state. After a while, you might have memorized it and you will begin to recognize and truly feel the natural abundance that is already within you. This is a powerful self-healing tool.

I am the sum total of my thoughts and beliefs
I forgive myself for the things I wish I had done differently
because I understand that I cannot change the past
From this day on I choose Inspiration
I choose Freedom, I choose Peace
I am grateful to Divine Intelligence which gives me the power
to smile at my weaknesses and utilize my potential
I welcome and accept the abundance that life has to offer
and I now know that I am worthy of it all
I feel contentment and deep gratitude to simply BE
Right Here, Right Now
I feel grounded and empowered as I acknowledge my needs
I am open to receiving the nourishment I deserve
I breathe in my own beauty
as I realize that I have been made to perfection
There is no one else who looks like me
Nobody else can live the life that was breathed into me
Or use the talent I was gifted with
I am deeply grateful to Divine Intelligence
I love and accept myself unconditionally as
I fully realize that I AM Source manifested
I am open to sharing Joy, Peace, and Laughter with loved ones
I surrender to life itself'

INTENTIONS: FRIENDS OR FOE?

Certainly, the revival of the law of attraction in getting what we desire has sparked everyone's interest. The mechanics of the law of attraction is, in the words of Abraham Hicks: "That, which you think, in any moment, attracts onto itself other thoughts that are like it". For the purpose of this book, however, I will only discuss this law with the aim of attuning to well-being physically, emotionally, mentally, and spiritually. Ultimately, what we intend for ourselves is never as expansive as what the Divine has in mind for us because it is the conscious, programmed mind that is making the requests, which is *always self-limiting.* We are *the manager* of our life and not *the owner,* as is commonly believed among adepts of the law of attraction. *The owner* is Divine Intelligence, which is inherent in each and every one of us.

Attention energizes and Intention transforms

Attention: What you *focus on* expands

- In negative terms, and to keep it simple, focusing on an illness, a debt, being overweight, or having a negative attitude will contribute to its expansion because this is accompanied by feelings that fuel thoughts into physical manifestation.
- In positive terms, the same is true of its opposite: feelings of strength, well-being, abundance, or belief in yourself will also contribute to more of the same in its expansion.

Intention: What you *intend on* transforms

Let me make something clear: there is no point in being in denial. I will use a financial example for just a second. If you are stone-broke, splashing out while affirming your wealth will not increase your bank balance! In other words, if you are in debt, a can of beans served on a slice of bread (eaten with gratitude) is definitely wiser than a lobster supper charged to your credit card!

You can *intend* on pulling yourself out of a particular situation by removing the inner resistance that keeps you out of the natural flow in your life. Vivid awareness enables you to recognize the next step to be taken or allows you to see an opportunity when it smiles at you, but you mustn't forget to acknowledge and surrender to the present moment and the situation as it is *first*. This keeps you clear of an inevitable inner struggle, which can otherwise become a stress and the antithesis to your well-being and natural abundance. If you do not surrender, you will find that further programming is cluttering your inner space, creating tremendous inner conflict as you strive to become something that you may not be ready for just yet. Any time you use the words *should* or *shouldn't*, you can pretty much bet that you are out of synch with the natural flow of your life, as you are putting attention on what *is not*.

Positive intentions are extremely powerful; they allow you to receive the necessary information for you to fall into synchronicity with your potential, but you must be easy about this. The ingredients to your success (whatever this may mean to you) have been there all along, but often remain invisible due to a restricted perception as the mind is cluttered with limited expectations. So the main intention that can allow your potential to shine through into complete abundance resides in your ability to remove personal resistances and outmoded negative beliefs. Ultimately, a lack of belief in yourself really means a lack of trust in the Source that created you ... something to overcome as soon as you can.

Note: For some fascinating research on the power of intentions, read Lynne McTaggart's book, *The Intention Experiment* (23).

Expansion beyond limited beliefs of hereditary illness and aging

The first step is to be able to accept that some of the beliefs you hold are limiting. It does not matter how true you think they are. In reality, they are only a collection of what you have heard and observed from others or research you have read. If illness or difficult aging is (or was) in your family, it can represent the environment that has formed your beliefs, and therefore dictate your personal expectations and have a considerable impact on your manifested reality. The only part of you that gets challenged by this idea, if you find this unsettling, is your ego, or conscious mind—which is made up of so many good reasons and excuses (with matching proofs!) on how things will go wrong because they did for your parents. These beliefs are only true if you let them be so.

Being at the mercy of limited beliefs also happens to people on their spiritual path who are already aware: *If you think* that you are free and are *feeling* ill or frustrated because your life is not reflecting what you know that it could, this is a sure indication that your mind is taking you for a ride and that you are letting it. The first step is to realize that you may not actually be as free as you thought, meaning that the pursuit of freedom can just be another trap (an elusive goal), or a new belief. Know this: there is no limit to your freedom and well-being, so it is best to keep that inner perception as open as can be!

The negative attention that perpetrates illness

Until now and for the most part, the intentions you have had are based on your past, your conditioning, your value system, and what you *expect* to be possible *for you*; in most cases, they are not very expansive. Most habits and beliefs are so deeply ingrained that you can find it extremely hard to do anything other than just *react* or *replay* until your awareness is vivid enough to recognize what is going on and wise enough to release the iron grip that is holding negative patterns, or so-called hereditary illness, firmly in place. The amount of programming is massive and plays into many areas of your life, but for now, let us just look at your health and your potential and see how you can become a *conscious participant* in your own existence, rather than a victim of outmoded beliefs.

There is plenty of scientific research today that clearly explains that hereditary illness is not as hereditary as we once thought, and that it is precisely the thoughts we entertain, followed by the emotional charge we carry, that determines how we age and dictates the state of our health. In other words, this is all up to you!

Note: What is discussed above is known as the science of epigenetics; if you would like to read a truly transformative book on this subject, I recommend *Molecules of Emotions* (25) by Candace B. Perth, Ph.D., neuroscientist.

Equally fascinating, cutting-edge research is described in *The Biology of Belief* (21) by Bruce H. Lipton, Ph.D., cell biologist.

Many people literally "nurse" a family pattern by reaffirming how inevitable its manifestation is for you. For example, let's say that your mother or father died of cancer or has Alzheimer's disease; your predetermination to something similar is very real, but only in as far as your chosen thoughts, which, if they are repetitive enough, can create matching emotions of fear and dread that bring manifested illness into your reality. Remember, *attention energizes*! It is really as simple as that.

In the direct opposite manner, this is the same reason that some people heal themselves after hearing they have contracted a deadly illness: they decide consciously, there and then in that moment, to pull themselves out of this unattractive predestined, only probable, reality. Remember, *energy follows thoughts, and intention transforms*! We call such instances miracles, and they can be performed by yourself, on yourself, anytime you notice you are holding a belief that is undeserving of who you really are.

The very same goes for aging; your preprogrammed expectations need to become clear to you, so you can transform them.

The Rejuvenating mind exercise

Simple exercise

Take a pen and a piece of paper and find a quiet and comfortable spot to sit. The aim of this exercise is to observe your belief system around aging and your health (your age is irrelevant here), so you can begin to transform what is not conducive to your natural abundance. Write down some key words or full phrases, and don't panic if it is really bad when you read it over; you can transform absolutely anything!

To me, aging means:

— …

— …

If you hold a lot of negativity around this natural process, see if you can identify where it originates (parents, media, outmoded medical research).

The origin of my belief is:

— …

— …

If you would like to experience change in your life, but feel unable to move past an "iron–clad" limited belief, use the following suggestions to help you identify your limitations:

- Does your current belief serve you in your life at present?
- If so, *how* does it serve you?
- Could you get a similar or even better result by changing your attitude?*

* For example, an unconscious motivation for "nursing" an illness and talking to friends and family about it can be rooted in the

attention you receive in the form of pity, which only breeds more of the same inside of you as self-pity. This form of attention-seeking can be transformed to a real sharing with loved ones, doing things you enjoy, which increases your well-being and extends your life expectancy.

My limiting beliefs are:

— ...

The acknowledgement of blockages, patterns, or limiting belief accounts for 90 percent of the work. The energy required to resolve any issue is 10 percent. In other words, all you really have to do for now is to observe your thought mechanism. This is easily done by staying alert, deciding that you want to age well, and having fantastic health. This decision need only be made once; everything else you may choose to do after that will feel like an inspiration and therefore will be fun and effortless. Isn't it time you started to live the life that was meant for you?

There are many methods that are helpful to shift limiting beliefs, EFT and NLP are two of them. Let us have a look at NLP.

NLP (Neuro-Linguistic Programming)

NLP provides tools and skills to help you move past limitations, accelerate personal growth, gain clearer vision, and open pathways so you can let your natural wisdom shine forth. It also helps you to gain access to personal competence on a worldly level so that you can excel at what you do. NLP highlights the workings of your mind and its multilevel ability to be at your service; you need not be at the service of your mind. Most people live like slaves, imprisoned by an incessant stream of thoughts, unable to feel the peace and joy within. NLP is one of many tools you might find beneficial in helping you to develop your potential.

NLP consists of the following:

N: *The neurological system* determines how your body functions according to your thoughts.

L: *The linguistic system* describes the relationship between the way you think and the language you use to communicate with the world.

P: *The programming* describes your behavioral patterns according to the above two principles. Simply stated, it determines how you bring about your reality.

Tip: Depending on the intensity of the results that you would like to achieve in your life, you might consider hiring a coach for accelerated personal success. Choose the right person according to the type of coaching you need, and make sure that you feel at ease with him or her. You need to be able to truly communicate if you are serious about removing obstacles and getting real results in your life.

Note: Anthony Robbins' book, *Unlimited Power* (26), is a wonderful tool and a catalyst in the understanding of how powerful you really are.

CAN YOU "ORDER" YOUR CELLS TO SELF-REGENERATE?

Yes! Or at least you can stay out of the way with negative beliefs. We have all heard of incredible cases where people heal themselves of cancer with sheer focus and determination. I propose *regeneration* and *self-rejuvenation* in the same line of thinking. Many people look *considerably* younger than their biological age; their *secrets* seem to be a combination of various factors:

- Having a positive outlook on life: you look relaxed when you feel relaxed!
- Being at peace and in tune with yourself: the most important relationship you'll ever get into
- Keeping informed/learning something new, challenging yourself
- Doing something you feel *true passion* for, whatever it might be!
- Feeling *real gratitude* for being here, now, as often as possible. Enjoying the immense gift that your life is
- Treating yourself as you would your best friend!

Rejuvenating meditation

I would like to invite you to practice this meditation which is designed with the aim of promoting complete cellular regeneration. This is also a good way to put yourself in an alpha state, also known as a meditative state, a great preparation before writing down your goals and feeling their manifestation coming into physical manifestation. This does not cost anything! We already know that *energy follows thoughts* and that cells renew themselves every second, so the following practice works in combining those facts to give you access to *complete holistic renewal.*

- While sitting comfortably on a chair or on the floor, put a hand on your heart.
- Feel the rhythm of your heart beating effortlessly, with natural intelligence.
- Feel the awesome gratitude for the life you have been given, for the magnificent body you inhabit.
- Let your gratitude radiate from your heart to every part of your body, like the sun rising and shining over the earth every day.
- When you feel an upsurge of joy and wellness, use your

breath to let it spread and permeate each and every organ, every cell, and every atom, and all the space in between.

- Feel yourself expanding, becoming limitless.
- Your nature is pure space, pure energy, pure potential waiting to be channeled into creation.
- Open your mind so you can receive inspiration and nourishment.
- Visualize your cells replicating themselves to the highest possible standard, feeding your subtle and physical systems with extra-ordinary strength and rejuvenating qualities.
- Quench your thirst by drinking from the source of everlasting life force.
- Give thanks with the knowledge that this energy is inherent in you, and available absolutely anytime you need or desire it.

Help yourself and assist the process by taking care of what you put into your body. A glass of crystal water would be a great complement to this ritual; see page 34 for more information. Any regular water will do if you don't have a crystal; just send it some loving thoughts before you drink it.

Rejuvenating bath

1. Run yourself a pampering bath with essential oils—woody scented oils like sandalwood and orange, for example, or rose and lavender, depending on your preference. Put a maximum of eight drops into a teaspoon of sweet almond oil, or 100 percent fat milk if that is all you have. The fat ensures that the essential oils are diluted and do not come into direct contact with your skin. Some people have very sensitive skin.
2. Yes, this is for you too gentlemen! You can also choose to

offer this bath-pampering ritual to your loved one—a beautiful gift.

3. You may add some flower petals, light some candles, and bring in a glass of wine or champagne.

Follow the same steps as the Rejuvenating meditation to do the rest of this ritual. See pages 237-238 for a list of rejuvenating crystals.

Note: The bath ritual offered here is great when shared with your partner. Any kind of prayer or meditation is amplified when two people express their needs for one another, and often manifest faster.

"When two people sit, God comes"

TOPICS EXPLORED IN SECTION 4

- Our basic functioning mechanism
- The power of creative potential
- Needs versus wants
- Gratitude Prayer
- Attention energizes and intention transforms
- Rejuvenating mind exercises
- Rejuvenating meditation
- Rejuvenating bath

NOTES

Chapter Four

UNUSUAL REJUVENATING SECRETS

1. Crystals

Crystals: A life-form that has inhabited the planet from its very beginning

They are a part of the earth's crust and are ancient tools, beautifully powerful and very much alive. Some people believe that they are a vestige of Atlantean technology. They are living entities with individual healing vibrational frequencies, powerful in their emissions which anyone or anything in their proximity can receive. This reaffirms the evidence that we are all intrinsically connected, and are therefore part of the whole. Crystals are used for many types of therapeutic and healing work, and they make beautiful healing jewelry. Larger crystal pieces can also be used at home or at the office; they assist in deflecting some of the negatives rays emitted by electronic equipment such as computers and TVs. They have been used in commercial applications for many years; most people are familiar with the presence of quartz in watches and in computers.

Note: As with a few other topics covered in this book, there are many more uses for crystals other than those discussed here, but we will only explore the stones that have detoxifying and rejuvenating properties.

If you would like to know more about the use of crystals, you will enjoy *The Crystal Bible* (16) by Judy Hall.

How do crystals work?

They emit a particular vibrational frequency, which was "imprinted" into their cellular makeup as they grew within the earth's crust. There are literally hundreds of different types of crystals, all absolutely fascinating. All crystalline structures are formed with Divine mathematical precision, which can be studied and is known as *sacred geometry*. Further studies show that such geometric patterns are in fact found in all Mother Nature's creations. The same patterns have been replicated and have served to inspire the blueprint on which sacred monuments and places of worship have been created since the beginning of time. We, human beings, were also designed by Divine Intelligence, originating from pure consciousness translated into vibrating atoms, molecules, cells tissues, which make up our organs and the rest of our body. Unfortunately, for the most part, we have forgotten who we are, and how connected we all are. Crystals have not. When we work with crystals, a simple interaction takes place: the innate healing vibration of the stone comes into contact with our auric field and reestablishes the harmony within. Different crystals carry different healing energies; some of them, such as quartz, can be programmed according to the individual's need, and all of them have regenerating properties.

Powerful tools

Although crystals are powerful tools, do not expect things to happen of their own accord, without your participation, as if "by magic." You need to open your mind and be reasonably focused to use any kind of new tool or approach, in this case working with crystals. Once you feel prepared to do a little fun work and experimentation, you can set out to find the crystal you need: the one that will work with you. Intention plays a *gigantic role* in working with crystals. If you want to get clear results, you need to give clear instructions; therefore your intentions need to be clean and precise. As discussed in the previous chapter, we have seen that *intention* is one of the main contributing factors with which you co-create your reality (23), in all areas of your life.

Myths about crystals

If you are familiar with crystals, you will probably have heard that you should never buy your own. This is not true at all. In fact, it is very important that you buy your own piece, as *you* need to be able to attune with it; otherwise it will not work. It is a little bit like a pair of shoes—they need to fit and feel comfortable; otherwise they will not be of any use! Having a crystal is like having a good friend, a relationship that started with a connection and some reciprocal energy. There is, however, an exception to this, which is that someone can pick a crystal for you, as long as she holds the definite *intention* of it being *for you*. So the attraction he or she feels when choosing a crystal piece holds you in mind.

For a number of years, as part of my former healing center, I ran a metaphysical shop selling crystals. I went on buying trips for the business, and some clients would request various kinds of pieces, some of them enormous geodes and collector's items. With their particular requests and uniqueness in mind, I scanned the place until I found a match for the client and the crystal. It never failed, not even once; the right crystals ended up meeting the right people, who were always grateful. This had nothing to do with me having super powers but simply an ability to "step aside" and let the energy guide me to bring home what that person needed. If I can do it, you can do it!

HOW TO CHOOSE YOUR OWN CRYSTAL

There are various ways of doing this and I will recommend a few here. If, however, you find other methods of choosing the crystal that is right for you, go ahead and do it your own way!

Your intuition is your best guiding force; don't ever let anybody or any books tell you otherwise; *you can rely on it fully*.

In-tuition = tuition from within.

On intuition ...

The seat of your intuition is not located around your heart or your head, as is commonly believed, but in your *solar plexus*. Whether you get excited on hearing good news or "get hit" with bad news, you usually feel it in your gut, which is why there is such a saying as your *gut feeling*. You can choose to ignore it, but it is always right. I call it the *inner compass:* very similar to an in-built GPS, something for which we can be immensely grateful. More often than not, the conscious mind will come in over a gut feeling and demand explanations for a seemingly irrational decision, only to find that if we had listened to our intuition, we would not have ended up in the predicament that we did. Indeed, the mind comes up with incredibly creative ways to make us doubt our inner guidance, which something to observe with vivid awareness! It takes a little practice to observe this inner conflict and to learn to differentiate between programmed mind patterns and intuition. With any of the methods offered below, it is important to feel relaxed, centered, and present in your own body. A deep breath always helps. It would also be a good thing for you to know *how* you take in your information, and *which* ways you best respond to different signals. Here are some tips.

ARE YOU A KINESTHETIC, AUDITORY, OR VISUAL PERSON?

If you are a kinesthetic person, your intuition guides you through your sense of touch. You need to *hold* the piece of crystal to find out *what feels right* for you. You can identify what you need through various *feelings* in your body, particularly your hands. A sensation of heat or cold, or "pins and needles" can sometimes be felt in your hand; or a wave of well-being can simply wash over you. Trust yourself to know when you are in touch with the stone you need. Alternatively, you can use your hand like a scanner by running it over a number of stones; make sure you take your time and stop over the piece that caught your *tactile* attention.

If you are an auditory person, your intuition guides you mainly through what you *hear*. Read the names of the stones aloud or ask a shop assistant to call out the crystals that are good for detoxification or cell renewal, for example, and trust your *auditory attraction* to indicate which one would work best with you.

If you are a visual person, you predominantly rely on what you *see* to find out what you like. Simply look around at all the crystals, and when you feel drawn to one, get closer and see if it appeals to you.

Tip: Besides crystal picking, the list above gives you valuable information to determine what your loved ones best respond to. You will be able to offer them gifts that will be much closer to their sensory delights!

Taking care of your crystal is very easy

Crystals are *beings*, and like any other living entity that can give and receive energy, they appreciate gratitude, respect, love, and care. When you first bring your stone home, you must cleanse it. Crystals record the energy of *everything and everyone* they have been in contact with; all information stays imprinted into it until it is cleansed. Don't worry, you will never be able to change its own healing programming by cleansing it. You just need to erase all unwanted influences.

Cleansing your crystal

There are various ways of cleansing your crystal, and again if you find your own technique, use that. Here are some guidelines:

- Hold it under cold running water for a few minutes while sending the *clear intention* that all unwanted influences must be cleansed.
- If you live by the sea, bring your crystal next time you go to the beach and bathe it with the same clear intention of purification. Running water like that of a river is also very cleansing.
- You can leave it in pure sea salt for two or three hours. Make sure the salt covers the stone and discard it when the job is done; it will have absorbed all the unwanted influences, none of which you want in your next meal!
- A lot of books on the subject advise using salted water overnight. I have found that this is not always wise as the stone may be mounted as jewelry, or it may be a softer type of crystal, in which case it can become corroded. If you want to use salted water, simply run the stone through it a few times. Do not let it soak.
- You can use sage smoke to "smudge" your stone. Originating from Native American tradition, this cleansing method is also great to cleanse people and places from negativity or blocked energy. Light up the sage bundle, blow out the flame, and fan the smoke toward the crystal. Be present, and hold your intention clear and focused.
- You can cleanse it with your own breath. Take a deep, conscious breath, making it your intention to purify the crystal, and simply exhale over it while staying focused. Repeat two or three times.

Note: Whichever method you choose, trust yourself to know when the cleansing is complete. There is no right or wrong amount of time to do this. The more you trust yourself, the more trust you will have in yourself.

Recharging your crystal

If your crystal feels, looks, or sounds seriously worn out, but you still bought it because you knew that it was the one for you, bury it in soil. Soil is the closest medium to its origin, so it works as a great purifier and cleanser, and it also gives your crystal a considerable boost. It does not need to be buried too deep; make sure you remember where you put it! If you find that it still needs to be recharged after two or three days, you can leave it in the soil for a few more days, or even for a few weeks if extremely depleted. I have seen very pale crystals regain their deep and vibrant colors after being recharged. Some stones have color in them, and some are transparent, like quartz. Don't worry, you will know when it feels better and when it is ready to use. How? Trust your intuition.

After the initial cleanse, all crystals need to be regenerated regularly, especially if you use them on a daily basis.

Here is what you can do:

- Leave it in sunlight for a few hours. The sunrays help realign the crystal's own light structure.
- Leave it in moonlight overnight; the same process will occur. For best night light, wait until the moon is at its fullest.

Using your crystal is easy

All crystals have their own particular healing frequency; so once cleansed, they are ready to use. Others can take extra programming, depending on your own particular requirements.

Clear quartz is a stone that you can program. After you have cleansed it, and before using it, ask your crystal *clearly* to help you with what you need. Be direct and precise in order to get direct and precise results. You basically need to talk to your stone as if you were asking a friend for help with a particular matter: be courteous and grateful!

- Hold the stone at gaze level, or press it gently against your forehead; it doesn't matter whether your eyes are open or closed, as the request will come from your third eye (the energy center situated between your eyes).
- Ask, "Dear crystal, I ask of you to assist me with ..." Wait a few moments; trust your intuition to know when it is programmed.
- Give thanks to your crystal.

This will become easier with regular practice. The more you see and feel the crystal energy working in your life, the easier it will be to connect with it, and the more powerful it will become. Talking to your crystal will become as normal as smiling down to your liver!

Tips on how to put your crystal to good use:

- Put it under your pillow before you go to sleep. You can ask it to help you with a good, rejuvenating night's sleep for example. You'll be pleasantly surprised by the results upon awakening!
- Most crystals are available as tumbled stones, which are soft all around, as they have been polished. Their energy may not be as strong as that of rough stones, but they are a wise choice if you are going to keep one on you. It can be put in a pocket, bra, etc. Handbags are too far from you to receive a small crystal's healing rays; so, for example, you could wear a tiny pouch hanging around the neck and under your clothes. Pendants and other jewelry items are also a good option to receive the healing rays of crystals.
- If it is a larger piece, place it near you: on your bedside table at night, in your car, on your desk, etc. Basically, keep it close to you, wherever you are.
- Crystals are also well known to absorb negative rays emitted by computers. For it to be effective, it would need

to be about the size of your fist (at least) and be on top of the monitor, or touching the laptop. It needs to be removed carefully with a cloth so you don't reabsorb the negative load that has been extracted and is now held in the crystal. Use a cloth to take it away and rinse your stone under running water for a little while. It will need a weekly recharge and cleansing. It can be used on television sets, Play Stations, or any other electrical equipment that is used for prolonged periods of time —basically all the electronic devices that give us "googly eyes" and extra frown lines!

- It can help to revive plants and trees that are feeling poorly. Simply put your crystal in the plant's soil until you notice a significant improvement. Natural quartz or rose quartz is best for that. If you have a pointed crystal, bury it into the soil pointing toward the root of the plant.
- You can put it in your bath, especially if your intent is to receive a healing or to have a detoxing and beautifying ritual bath. Be careful if the stone is sharp that you don't cut yourself.
- It can be used to increase the potency of any of your beauty products, particularly if they are made with natural essential oils like the creams and lotions on pages 100-102. Simply place it under the product overnight. This also works to greatly regenerate any foodstuff.

Crystal elixirs have been used since the beginning of civilization; they offer another simple and efficient way to absorb the energy from your crystal. There is no side effect to using crystals; the worst thing that can happen is that it might not work, which would only be because your mind is closed. Don't forget that your intention is your most influential factor—whether it is negative or positive, you are always right ... the choice is yours!

How to make your elixir:

- Find a glass or a pottery jug; avoid plastic, as some of its molecules inevitably transfer into the water.
- Put your crystal in water and leave it for a couple of hours. Water is a natural conductor of energy, so it will take on the vibration of the crystal.

If you would like to store your elixir for long periods of time, find a glass bottle and mix in some brandy (about 30 percent) to give it a longer shelf life. Anytime you need to use it, simply add a few drops of the elixir to a glass or a bottle of water.

Uses of crystal elixir:

- Wash your face or make a facial mist; leave out the brandy in this case!
- A nice way to use crystals for the whole family (including pets) is to put a piece of quartz in a water jug and leave it there permanently. Rinse it from time to time to make sure that it does not accumulate slime, and charge it regularly, e.g., once a week. Clear quartz restores your tap water's natural life force, which is important, as it goes through lengthy treatments and filtering to become drinkable.
- If some of your plants are looking like they could do with a boost, and the crystal planted in the soil doesn't work fast enough to repair the damage done, use crystal water to feed it and you are certain to see prompt regeneration take place.

You may wonder what the plants have to do with rejuvenating properties. Keep reading into the next section on Plants to give yourself a better understanding of how connected everything really is.

List of beautifying crystals:

The following listed crystals are good for cell and tissue

regeneration; they contribute to the elimination of toxins in the body and the mind. They are particularly rejuvenating when the elixir is used on the skin and taken in water:

- Quartz, rutilated quartz, and rose quartz
- Peridot
- Topaz
- Selenite (also protects and rejuvenates male sexual glands)

Note: Using one crystal from this list is enough. I am giving you a selection to choose from, though; there is never any harm in using a few if you would like to do that.

2. Plants

Plants, bountiful gifts from nature

Whether at home or at work, they make a healthy and visually pleasing addition to any environment. Luscious plants not only give "life" to their surroundings, but they also ensure that you breathe in good, organically recycled air. They transform carbon dioxide, water, and light into precious oxygen. Most modern houses and offices are like sealed containers nowadays, so well insulated that there is no air flowing; nothing gets in *or* out! This has given rise to a large amount of allergies, feelings of tiredness, lack of focus, and proliferation of airborne germs.

At home

Certain synthetic materials used in the building and decorating of a modern house can eventually have a taxing effect on our intricate biosystems. Smoke and cooking vapors pollute the air, so having plants in your living area is very important and considerably more pleasant than using synthetic air-fresheners. There are thousands of beautiful plants to choose from that are very easy to care for. Just make sure you get the necessary advice when you buy them to ensure that you are placing them in a favorable area of your house, garden, or balcony. You want your plants to be happy so they can be lush and vibrant with life force.

Plants for the bedroom

As you probably already know, most plants produce oxygen in the daytime and recycle their carbon dioxide at night. This is why you may have often heard that you should not keep any plants in your bedroom: so you don't absorb toxicity while you sleep. There are exceptions to this rule, however—plants that function in the opposite way, expelling carbon dioxide in the daytime, thus making them a valuable addition to your sleeping space. You'll be inhaling first-hand oxygen while you sleep and awaken feeling rested and looking refreshed by morning time.

Some of these plants are:

- Fittonia verschaffeltii (also known as snake skin plant)
- Aloe vera barbadensis

There are many types of aloe plants; the variety mentioned here can also be used for sun and first-degree burns. Aloe is a companion well worth having in several spots at home; an extra plant on the windowsill of your kitchen will prove useful for emergency kitchen burns. Simply squeeze a little juice from one of the leaves onto the burned skin. Again, treat your plant as the living being that it is. Ask the plant for its permission before cutting off a piece of the leaf and be suitably grateful for its healing properties once you feel better. Recycle the remains of the leaf by burying it in its own soil.

Note: I have read some research on plants stating that they cannot release oxygen unless there is a source of light in the room. While I am not absolutely sure about that point, a low consumption 5-amp green-energy bulb may be used in the bedroom.

Tip: Plants can transform a desolate balcony or a barren garden into a little place of heaven. If you don't have a lot of room for planting, there is always the option of keeping them in pots. You will benefit doubly if you cultivate aromatic herbs, as you will be able to use them to make teas or add flavor to your dishes. And let's face it: there is a certain degree of satisfaction that comes from knowing that you grew your own herbs to make fragrant teas and delicious salads! Watch what you spray on the leaves for bugs; stay organic.

Green roofs, also known as "eco roofs," are a superb growing trend which is beneficial for the environment and therefore for us too. I love them because they remind us that we are all interconnected, all part of an intricate eco-system. Green roofs are suitable for private houses almost anywhere, including in cities and on top of hotels, businesses, etc. There are literally gardens planted on an eco roof; read *Green Roof Plants: A Resource and Planting Guide* (30) by Edmund and Lucie Snodgrass.

3. Amaroli, or "Elixir of Life"

Are you ready to be challenged?

Then allow me to rattle your reason and challenge your belief system a little! You may or may not have heard of urine therapy before; if this is the first time you are hearing about it, it will probably shock you a little. Your mental perception is definitely being challenged; years of set beliefs have erected strong psychological barriers that can trigger a mental or a physical rejection of trying this method, or even reading about it! This practice requires a desire to explore your own healing potential and develop trust in your inner guidance. The benefits of amaroli (Indian name for urine therapy) are so rejuvenating that I could not leave it out of this manual. The following is for the courageous reader only!

A little history on amaroli

There is actually nothing new about the use of urine as a healing remedy. It has been used for thousands of years and has simply been forgotten as more sophisticated solutions have been developed. Of course, amaroli is not a "cure all"; nothing ever is. Each method is best kept for certain conditions, and not everybody can benefit from it. A lot of "age-old remedies" have been brought to our attention by resurfacing in the general public's interest, and they often tend to go through a fad stage, where they are overused for anything and everything. I think that it is reasonable to assume that no such thing will happen with urine therapy! It is used by a minority of people, but the ones who do use it are the grateful beneficiaries of *powerful rejuvenating benefits*.

Another name for the use of urine is Shivambu. It originated in India and was used 2,600 years ago by the Buddha and his disciples to cleanse their body and mind, and keep their spirit connected to the Source. It was believed, and still is by those who practice it, that drinking one's own urine keeps the body young, strong, and vibrant.

General uses for amaroli

Amaroli can assist the body to heal and repair itself with great success. It has been used and studied by qualified practitioners to treat a wide range of diseases, from skin ailments such as eczema to more serious illnesses such as cancer. Urine notably contains the hormone melatonin, which is responsible for keeping the stress levels down, and is instrumental in disabling the development of cancer cells.

Note: For more research and study on this topic, read *The Water of Life* by John W. Armstrong (4) and *The Golden Fountain* by Coen van der Kroom (19).

Personal experiences with amaroli

- I coached several clients to treat themselves with their

own urine for a wide range of skin complaints. They had positive and permanent results, much to their surprise!

- I used it to get rid of impetigo on my own children when they were very young. Impetigo has the reputation of being very hard to eliminate, as it is highly contagious—a nightmare if you have a few children, as it can go around the family for quite some time. The impetigo took an absolute maximum of three weeks to be eliminated permanently, which is hard to match with any other remedies or allopathic medicine currently available.
- I travelled India for many years and used my own amaroli instead of inoculations and malaria tablets. I never got sick.
- I use it to this day for a few weeks at a time; it is *the best anti-wrinkle product on the planet,* and IT'S FREE!

Note: Check the contraindications below before you use your own amaroli for anything at all. If you are considering using this method for anything other than rejuvenation, make sure that you talk to someone who practices this therapy professionally. Get onto the Internet and look for a urine therapy practitioner. The book recommended here (19) is very useful. Once again, the suggestions made below are for cosmetic purposes only.

What is urine exactly?

Urine is in fact filtered blood, and not a waste product that is dirty, as we have been raised to believe. It is a perfectly sterile substance and is composed of 95 percent water, 2.5 percent urea, and 2.5 percent mineral salts, enzymes, and hormones. Urea can be dangerous, but only if directly absorbed into the bloodstream in large quantities.

- The unborn child floats in amniotic fluid, which consists mainly of urine, while he/she develops. Doctors have also found that operations performed on unborn children during the mother's pregnancy leave no scars.

- You will have heard, no doubt, about soldiers in the war who urinated on their wounds to disinfect themselves.
- There are also a number of reports about people who were trapped in conditions where they had no access to food or drink. They used their own urine as the only means of survival available and came out of the experience in surprisingly good condition.

Tip: If you are ever stranded on your own somewhere with nothing to eat or drink, you know what to do! If you are ever stranded somewhere with people, drinking your urine is definitely easier than eating your friends.

Urea present in beauty products?

Yes, that is right. In fact, this is old news, as our Egyptian ancestors already used their own water for its rejuvenating and regenerative properties. Have you never noticed *urea* on labels of cosmetic creams? Look again next time you go shopping for costly moisturizers ... my suggestion is: if you are going to use urea, it might as well be your own! Urea has a great effect on cell regeneration and makes the skin soft and supple. It is not only absolutely free but is also the best prescription for beauty you will ever find, as it is completely tailor-made ... and it really works! Some actors and actresses (no names will be mentioned here) are well known to use their own urine every morning to maintain their youthful looks and vibrant health.

Preparing to use your own water

Some important facts are to be taken into consideration, such as food and drinks intake. The urine will taste a lot stronger if the food ingested makes it taste so.

Avoid the following if you are considering trying this method:

- Tea and coffee
- Alcohol and tobacco

- Allopathic and recreational drugs
- Bad fats (frying, using too much butter and margarine)
- Meat and fish

Note: Meat and fish may be eaten occasionally, like once or twice per week at the most, but you should make sure that it is organic. Anything nonorganic is treated with all sorts of chemicals that you definitely do not want to reabsorb.

All the above foods and drinks will make the urine taste very strong and bitter, therefore hard to take, and in some cases unsafe to drink. Another benefit to using your own water is that it motivates you to eat healthy food. When you eat wholesome food, your urine is lighter and has very little taste, almost like a light broth. As you start to feel and look better, it works as a natural incentive to treat yourself with more respect. Your daily habits become more favorable toward supporting your new choices, and this can have a rippling effect on other areas of your life. When you start to take control of your life, you are less likely to fall back into the old addictions and patterns that hold you prisoner.

Understanding that you can be self-sufficient in resolving a large number of your own issues with your own tools is very empowering

Tips: If you go to a party or a celebration where you eat rich food and/or drink alcohol, simply skip the next day's amaroli.

If you take herbs or vitamins, you will be reabsorbing a small amount of it, which may in fact be beneficial, although it can make the urine a little stronger. Make sure that the vitamins you buy are extracted from natural sources only; health food stores offer a good range.

How to use your own precious water:

Once you get over the initial reflex of disgust, you will find that your own water is indeed very pleasant to use. It has a rich, grainy quality to it (unlike water) and when rubbed onto the skin as a beautifying elixir, it gives an immediate glow.

- The best urine to use is fresh and midstream. Catching it midstream will eliminate the presence of residues from the urinary canal.
- You can use it neat on your face, around the eyes, on your neck, and of course anywhere on your body. Rinse after ten to twenty minutes. Use your moisturizer as usual.
- If you want to drink it, you don't have to take very much at all to begin with; a homeopathic dose of two or three drops in a glass of juice can be a good starting point.
- If you decide to drink it neat, a few sips are fine until you are able to drink a full glass. When taken by the glass, some people experience a healing crisis—meaning that an old ailment resurfaces to be cleansed out, usually once and for all.
- If you have scalp problems or your hair is thinning, use it as a lotion to massage your head. Rinse it off after about fifteen minutes. It will have had time to be absorbed into your scalp and hair, which will be left in superb condition: soft and shiny!
- It is also very effective as an aftershave. Rinse after ten or twenty minutes and put on some scented moisturizer if you think that you can still smell it. Be reassured that it is only *a thought (psychological smell!)* if you smell it after you have rinsed your face.
- You can use your own urine for a few weeks at a time—one or several times a year. If you are serious about a cure of holistic rejuvenation, a few months or a full year will yield brilliant results.

Important considerations

You have probably been raised to believe that urine is horrendous waste, so be gentle and patient with yourself if you are considering using it. The process you will have to go through to deprogram your mind might take a little while, which is normal. You are undoing a lifetime of very set beliefs. Inform yourself as much as you can and read about other success stories; this will help.

I remember the first time I decided to drink it; I felt consciously open and ready to try it and had many chats with my belief system. I took my first sip and the minute it reached my stomach, it came speeding back up. Although *I felt* absolutely ready, my subconscious mind overrode the decision and provoked my physical body to reject it. It took another few days before my body could keep it down. I prefer to take it in homeopathic doses, which is just as effective and much easier to drink.

Tips: If you cannot drink it neat, you can take your urine in homeopathic dosages. That means that you only use a few drops, so you won't taste it *at all*. Simply put five to six drops in a glass of juice. You will still get very good results this way. You may wish to increase your dosage once you get used to the idea and once you have adjusted your diet. Fresh, healthy urine is very clear and does not smell of anything in particular.

CONTRA-INDICATIONS

People who have serious medical conditions should not use this method, as they are probably taking some allopathic medicine.

People who have kidney, urinary or bladder, infections should not use this method at all.

TOPICS EXPLORED IN CHAPTER 4

- The use of crystals as personal tools
- Choosing and cleansing your crystal
- What is your main mechanism of perception?
- Rejuvenating crystal elixir
- Do you have green plants in your house?
- Green roofs for planet rejuvenation
- The use of amaroli for complete rejuvenation

NOTES

Chapter Five

COSTLY REJUVENATING SECRETS

1. Teeth and Hair

TEETH

Take a bite out of life

Teeth are nice when they are well taken care of and in good health. The alignment does not seem to matter so much, as long as they are a reasonably healthy color. There are plenty of whitening toothpastes to choose from, which can be misleading. The problem with most is that they basically scratch the enamel, giving the illusion of whiter teeth for a brief period of time. The next time you have tea, coffee, a glass of red wine, or a cigarette, the stains reappear, often darker than ever. Talk to your dentist if you want to use a whitener; ask him/her to recommend a brand of toothpaste that is effective and cleanses the teeth without harsh abrasion.

Laser whitening is very effective when done by a reputable dentist. It brings back the color of your teeth to their original shade. The procedure is painless and takes about an hour. Following this initial cleanse, you can purchase a professional kit (from your dentist) to keep your teeth white, to be used as a top-up treatment every six months or so. The dentist will take an imprint of your teeth and create a mold just for you. Too much polishing is not good, as it is eventually corrosive. Naturally white teeth look really nice, there is no need to expect snow white teeth as it might not suit your face and can look quite unnatural. Super-bright white teeth can be a little disturbing if they upstage your general presence!

Tip: If you need to brighten up your smile for an emergency date or a job interview, you can use strawberries. This *must not* become a habit, as the acid rubbed directly onto your teeth will eventually damage the enamel.

Strawberry dental spread

1. Crush one strawberry.
2. Mix with one-half teaspoon of baking soda.
3. Spread onto teeth with a soft toothbrush (soft brushes are *always* a better option to avoid causing gums to recede),
4. Leave on for five minutes.
5. Brush your teeth with regular toothpaste and floss to remove seeds in between teeth!

HAIR

We are blessed with hair dyes that can take years off the appearance of our face

This is accessible to most people, as many good dyes are available for home use. Let us not forget that gray hair can be very beautiful if the person wears it well, with self-confidence and dignity. This is very much a matter of preference.

Not ready for grays?

Dyes are an absolute blessing, as hair makes a huge difference in your overall appearance. Proceed with caution when choosing a hair dye; make sure the color works to enhance your looks. You might benefit from seeking help and advice from a professional hairdresser, at least for the first time you use hair dye.

Here are a few tips to look your best:

- Beware of overusing hair dye at home; the hair eventually becomes heavily coated with product, which can look very unnatural.
- Men and women past a certain age (up to you to decide which) should use very dark dye cautiously. It can give an overly severe appearance which, in some cases, can even look scary. Highlights are a good choice for a lot of people, as they can look very natural when well done. They are great to disguise the first few white hairs discreetly.
- If you are a man who dyes your hair, most women will tell you this: keep the salt-and-pepper look, at least around the temples. It gives a look of charm, distinction, and maturity, which is attractive!
- We all want to look our best—and very often, less is more.

A bald head can be attractive; I can think of many bald men who are striking. If there are still a few areas of hair on the head, the condition can be a little more delicate for the owner, it seems. In reality, of course, being bald (partly or fully) is not an issue at all if one has self-confidence. The worse disguise apparatuses are probably the "toupee" or the "comb-over." These look awfully obvious and are *almost never* perceived as sexy by anybody (except perhaps for Mr. Donald Trump!). And think of this: what will happen if you are caught in a strong gust of wind or are in the throes of passion with your loved one? Better to have a solid sense of humor!

Tip: If there are a few patches of hair left on the head, a good option can be to simply shave off the rest and be *beautifully bald.*

Is there a magical treatment for hair loss?

If a person has observed baldness in the family and baldness has occurred for him or her, it is reasonable to assume that it will not be remedied naturally. There are no products available anywhere on the market today that will make hair regrow in such cases. Why not consider the use of hair implants if the loss of hair causes you to be seriously distressed? It would be fair to say that if you look well (you already do, but let's say in your own opinion), you feel well; and if you feel well, you perform better in all areas of your life because you feel more self-confident. We are privileged to live in an era where such a choice is available, so why not allow yourself to do it if it is important to you?

Possible exceptions

Hair loss (alopecia) originating from emotional stress, chemotherapy, hormonal changes due to pregnancy, and certain illnesses linked to thyroid function can be remedied. In those few cases, it is possible and reasonable to expect the hair to grow back. Try the natural methods offered in this book (or any others you may find) for a period of time before making a decision regarding more drastic measures.

Tips: Regular and vigorous scalp massage is important while washing the hair or scalp, as it encourages local blood circulation and therefore increases the volume of oxygenated blood around the hair follicles, which can encourage growth. The very best essential oil you can use is rosemary; simply add two or three drops to your shampoo for one treatment. Use the most natural shampoo you can find; you don't want anything loaded with chemicals, as this will negate the delicate properties of essential oils. If you have so little hair that you cannot wash it, use a little sweet almond oil mixed with two-thirds of a drop of rosemary essential oil. Massage into the scalp up to twice a day.

A happy client

I once treated a young girl here, in Ireland, who suffered from alopecia due to a lengthy and particularly stressful time in her life. She, in fact, had lost most of her hair and was doubly distressed by this new symptom. I made up a prescription for her with some natural essential oils and vitamins, to be massaged onto her head daily. When the hair started to grow back, I used the same ingredients in a natural shampoo base, which she used whenever she washed her hair. It took three months for *all her hair* to grow back, and when it did, it grew in even thicker than before she had lost it. Mother and daughter came back to share their gratitude with a smile brighter than sunrise.

Caution: Refrain from using rosemary essential oil in the evening, as it is extremely stimulating on the central nervous system and may stop you from falling asleep; conversely, it works wonders if you need to study or drive late at night. People who suffer from epilepsy or pregnant women should not use rosemary oil, as it is too stimulating.

HAIR IMPLANTS

Hair implantation is the last resort, and it is expensive. As with all cosmetic surgery procedures, it is better to discuss the matter with a qualified and experienced professional before making any decisions. However, it gives great results, as it offers the most permanent intervention for hair loss known to date.

Follicular hair transplant is a minor surgical procedure performed over the course a few hours. A local anesthetic is administered while the surgeon obtains hair from the side and the back of the head, also known as the *donor area*. This is the hair in that area is genetically programmed to grow for life, so it will carry on growing naturally. The hair from the donor area is separated into individual follicles, which is then transplanted to the required area. The surgeon literally performs a work of art, meticulously spreading the new hair to resemble natural growth—a lengthy and delicate process, which explains the cost of the operation. One thousand grafts are transplanted over a four-hour period. If another treatment is required, the client will be advised to return for further surgery at a later stage. Regular hair care such as washing and cutting can resume shortly after this procedure, and no special maintenance is required.

Side effects can include swelling, itching, crust formation, and bruising around the eyes; but they all disappear within a few days or weeks.

Tip: Arnica pills can be taken to decrease the swelling and bruising, before and after treatment.

TOPICS EXPLORED IN SECTION 1

- Make the most of your teeth
- Baldness, hair dyes, toupees, and comb-overs!
- Tips to promote thick and beautiful hair
- Hair implants and tips for recovery

NOTES

2. Botox and Restylane

A WORD ON COSMETIC PROCEDURES

Treatments such as Botox and face fillers such as Restylane or Sculptra were once available to a select few only. Nowadays, they are both widely available to the general public, and have grown in popularity to such an extent that they are called "lunchtime procedures." The prices charged are relatively high, but not so much so that they are not accessible to most. Both treatments are used by men and women alike. Most doctors use Botox to eliminate the appearance of superficial wrinkles, and Restylane to fill deeper creases. It is very important to select a qualified and experienced doctor or nurse before getting anything done to your face. Usually, only doctors are trained to administer Botox; it is illegal for nurses to dispense Botox in the United Kingdom and Ireland. There are many nurses who are extremely skilled in the use of so-called fillers such as Restylane, Sculptra, and Juvederm. Please note that lip and cheek augmentation almost always look "done" in male clients. As with most cosmetic procedures, there may be side effects after a treatment has been received, so we will discuss them and explore valuable tips in individual sections a little further on.

If you choose to go ahead with either treatment, make sure you proceed consciously (and cautiously) after considering the benefits, risks, expense, and possible side effects. Once you have all the facts at your disposal, you can make better choices. Ask yourself if this is really what you want, because the word "need" does not even come into the picture here; there is nothing necessary about either, or any of the following procedures. Do not let any cosmetic treatments *replace the Secrets* we have explored in the first four chapters to keep yourself looking and feeling great; such tradeoffs do not work in the long run!

However, cosmetic enhancements such as Botox, or the judicious use of fillers, can make a huge difference to your external appearance in just a couple of hours. Treatments need to be maintained by a committed client and a cautious and competent doctor. All these procedures are reversible and look best on someone who is also living well, in every sense of the word. See all the other *secrets* offered in Chapters One, Two, Three, and Four.

WRINKLE BUSTERS

BOTOX, or Botulinum toxin type A is a highly purified derivative of a toxin that could be hazardous in much larger doses (2,500–3,000 units).

A normal dosage for cosmetic use would range between 10 and 20 units per area applied. Pregnant or breastfeeding women should stay away from such a procedure in case of possible side effects to their infants.

Botox was discovered by accident in the 1980s, when researchers stumbled upon its relaxing effects on muscle spasms associated illnesses such as cerebral palsy. It was also approved and used within a few years for the rectification of "crossed eyes" and "involuntary winking." An ophthalmologic doctor noted that the sites surrounding the injections were smoother after a treatment; the wrinkles were disappearing! Within another short few years, a medical paper was written by cosmetic dermatologists, and Botox was born as the most efficient wrinkle buster of all times.

Botox is also one of the most effective allopathic treatments for profuse axillary sweating. This condition is called hyperhidrosis, and can be a devastating social handicap for many people. The doses required are five to six times those of cosmetic treatments, and are injected into the skin of the affected armpit. It is very effective and can last up to six months at a time.

Precaution before a Botox treatment

Stop taking aspirin a couple of days prior to Botox, as it will increase the possibility of excessive bruising at the site of the injection. If you are on medication of any kind or need to take the aspirin daily, check with your GP before having anything done.

Tips: Take arnica, which is a homeopathic remedy for hematoma (bruising) just before and after the treatment if you bruise easily. You can take one pill up to every two hours the first day, and two or three times throughout the next day if you are badly bruised. Arnica pills or cream are available in most pharmacies and health food stores. You can also use arnica cream applied topically; the arnica gel is too strong if used close to the eye. Many people find that bruises subside faster with arnica and some report no improvement whatsoever. You'll have to try it yourself to see if it works for you, but make sure you *keep an open mind*—it will work better!

Note that when you take a homeopathic pill, to ensure its maximum benefit, do not handle it directly but use the lid to transfer it to your mouth. Let it dissolve under the tongue until fully melted for best results. Avoid coffee, smoking, and peppermint toothpaste while using homeopathy; these can negate the effect of arnica. The bruising, if any, is only minor and should disappear within a few days.

Precautions after a Botox treatment

You must avoid vigorous exercise, particularly up-down movements such as treadmill use, kneeling down for long periods, and lying down for a few hours after a treatment. Any sweating or rubbing on the area treated with Botox might interfere with the placement of the injection and produce side effects. Some doctors also advocate that you not get your hair washed (or wash your own) after a treatment, and not embark on a long flight.

Side effects of Botox

Although rare occurrences, you may experience headaches,

drooping of the eyebrow and/or eyelid, or double vision after an injection of Botox. Most side effects range from unnoticeable to a droop that is obvious and takes up to six weeks to disappear. Ask your doctor to explain these effects clearly to you, and check what percentage of their clients has suffered a "frozen brow or eyelid." Some doctors advocate the use of Iopidine eye drops, which can improve the appearance of the asymmetry, but does not make it disappear any earlier. Such side effects can be caused by a large amount of Botox being injected in a particular area. Or the doctor may not be qualified or experienced enough, *which is something you want to avoid at all costs.* Word of mouth is the best and safest way to find a reputable practitioner in your area. Always check their qualifications and never be afraid to ask questions; you are the client and you are trusting this person to perform a minor surgery on your face! At times, you may be responsible for the drooping if you rubbed the treated site shortly after the injection, thereby displacing the product. Lying down after a treatment is not recommended either for the same reason. The long terms side effects of Botox are not known, as it has only been used for a relatively short time.

Note: At the risk of repeating myself, I will say again that checking in first with your inner guidance is always important, particularly before going ahead with any procedures. Your instinct is always right, so trust it. If you have any doubt, you might be wise not to go ahead with it for now. *Doubt means no.*

The benefits of Botox

When Botox is applied successfully, you look well rested and refreshed, as if you had a good night's sleep or a holiday. Some of the tension is gone from the face; however, the treatment should not block *all* facial movements, which can look a bit strange and terribly obvious. Botox is generally used for the top half of the face: around the eyes, between the eyebrows, and on the forehead. The results can be a dramatic improvement of the skin, which becomes smoothed out and wrinkle-free. Final results can take anything from three to ten days. The effect of the treatment can last between three or four months before wrinkles slowly come back in a very progressive way.

Note: For best results with Botox, there must be a certain amount of elasticity in the skin. Men and women with deep lines and/or very loose skin may not see any improvement from Botox. Other treatments such as skin peels, a facelift, or a thread-lift may be undertaken if deemed necessary. Alternatively, enjoying life and developing a sense of deep gratitude (and surrender) may be what you need most! See the Gratitude Prayer on pages 215-216.

When is the best time to start using Botox?

This is very much up to you, but there is no need to start too early. Bear in mind that the skin starts aging noticeably around 35, a reasonable time to start using a little Botox. Very little can be done for the neck area, so make sure you moisturize it as often as possible. Some Botox can be injected in that area but the risks are very serious (ranging from altered voice to an inability to swallow), so good sense should prevail against accepting such risks. In much older people, the face can sometimes look too young against an older neck, which can look a little odd. At some point, it may be more gracious to give up using cosmetic procedures altogether.

Using Botox is great to freshen up the face, and don't forget that it looks best when you keep a few natural lines. A permanently frozen expression is never natural looking, so use it sparingly for best results!

Botulinum creams and gels

There is no evidence that Botox topical products are absorbed through the skin and no study has shown that these creams, gels, or lotions are effective. These creams were developed targeting people who do not want to receive injections but still want to have smoother skin. The cost of these topical treatments is not a lot less than Botox injections—and they produce no noticeable effects.

FACIAL FILLERS

Restylane and Perlane

Both of these products are in fact hyaluronic acids. Hyaluronic acid is a polysaccharide, or natural sugar, that is present in the human body where it plays a crucial role by contributing to cell growth and keeping the skin plump and supple. Restylane has the capacity to bind to water many times its volume. In some countries, the type of hyaluronic acid (collagen) used is still extracted from animal sources, but the risk of infection is so much higher that it is better to use a synthetic filler: the two brands discussed here are manmade in laboratories. There is no allergy test required, as the risk of reaction is minimal. Both fillers have a similar composition, although one is thicker than the other. Your cosmetic doctor decides which to use based on the thickness of your skin and the depth of the wrinkle that needs to be filled. The product is injected directly into the upper layers of the skin, usually around the lips to minimize "bleed-lines," into the lips for plumping effects, and into the nasolabial folds, or to fill up unsightly scars. It is mainly used on the bottom part of the face, although some adventurous doctors can sculpt cheekbones and chins. For the most part, though, it is used to fill up lines and scars. A local anesthetic is used in the form of an injection and/or a topical cream before the filler is administered. There are new products coming out all the time, so make sure you do a little research, as I cannot cover everything here.

Precautions before fillers

These are quite similar to the Botox recommendations. Do not take aspirin, as it thins out the blood and can increase the risk of severe bruising at the injection site. Again, arnica taken just before the treatment and up to a few days afterward can be very helpful (see notes for Botox).

Side effects

There can be some serious bruising and swelling at the site of filler injections, particularly when used to augment lips or cheeks. Keep taking arnica pills every two hours if necessary, and apply arnica cream or gel directly on the skin that has been treated. Alternatively, dilute one drop of lavender essential oil in a little moisturizing base cream (or aloe vera gel) and apply every two hours. Lavender is anti-inflammatory as well as being extremely soothing, and it works very well to fade bruises.

Tips:

- Eat a small amount of freshly cut pineapple if you are bruised. This is very useful after any cosmetic treatments or *any other surgical operation* when there is bruising to the skin. It assists the healing process in several ways: it contains an enzyme called bromelain, which dramatically helps to fade any bruising, and vitamin C, which contributes considerably to tissue repair.
- Pineapple is a super-food and a powerful antioxidant; it also has anti-inflammatory properties, so it is great for any swelling.
- *Buy natural pineapple;* the canned version has little or no vitamins left and is particularly lacking in bromelain, which you need most.

Note: Pineapple is also useful for sprains and strains.

Side effects of fillers

There is a small possibility that some of the injected product can cause a local infection, which can materialize as a raised area under the skin. Professional cosmetic doctors use an antiseptic cream on the injection site as soon as all the work is completed.

You can ask for some antiseptic cream to take home, or get a prescription if a local infection occurs after an injection. It should disappear within a few days, but if it is pronounced, it may remain for a number of weeks.

If you are prone to bruising in general, anticipate that you will most probably get a few bruises, so avoid business lunches and romantic dates straight after your cosmetic treatment. You will be quite red where the work was done, but this can be covered with a little concealer; and it fades quickly. You are now well equipped to deal with your side effects when you get home. All bruises should disappear in a matter of days with the tips recommended here. Fillers are a relatively new procedure, so there is no research on the long-term side effects.

Do yourself a favor: Help yourself!

Especially if you have just invested some money and put up with some pain and few bruises to get this done: DRINK SOME WATER! Now that you know what those fillers are made of, and that they bind to water, it would be a shame not to help yourself. Enough water drunk daily will extend the life span of your fillers and keep your skin in top condition (see page 29 for information on water intake). Also, some of the lines you may be trying to fill up may be due to premature aging linked to smoking, so you know what to do.

The benefits of fillers

Those deep creases have disappeared and your face now looks plumped up. The effects can last between six and twelve months. Be discreet about your use of fillers: a large quantity can make the face too puffed up and, in some unfortunate cases, a little bit like a chipmunk's! We have all seen people who have abused cosmetic procedures on TV or in magazines, and it really is not very attractive. Used discretely, fillers can help you keep your natural, youthful appearance for a few more years.

When is the best time to start using fillers?

This is up to you of course but once again up to your own discretion. Bear in mind that they are used to fill up deeper creases, so maybe you should wait until they begin to appear. Prevention of wrinkles is best achieved with some of the information included in the first three chapters. You won't see any serious lines or deep creases appear on your face before the ages of thirty-five to forty.

TOPICS EXPLORED IN SECTION 2

- History and uses of Botox and face fillers
- Side effects of Botox and face fillers
- Tips for prompt and easy recovery before and after cosmetic interventions

NOTES

3. Skin Resurfacing and Chemical Peels

SKIN RESURFACING

Does that sound like road works?

Yes? Well, this is probably because it is a little like road works! It is basically taking away the upper layer of the skin (the epidermis), so that it can renew itself, free from blemishes. Some treatments reach the deeper layers of the dermis, depending on the results required. The after-effects and the results can both be quite imposing, with a lengthy recuperation time in some cases. People with sensitive skin may not benefit from such methods, as the side effects and the amount of time invested may be too high a price to pay.

There are all sorts of skin resurfacing methods available, but I would highly recommend that you *only go* to a doctor who will explain clearly *all* the possible side effects for each treatment available. Another thing to bear in mind is that the kind of peel available to you depends on your skin type, the thickness of your skin, and the current state that it is in. Make sure you gather all the information you need before committing to a treatment. Ask what the best procedure would be *for you*; express your desires and expectations *clearly*. The more informed you are, the better and more empowered choices you can make.

If you are looking to get rid of some wrinkles and creases, Botox and/or face fillers would be more effective. Skin resurfacing is usually best suited to improving the texture and quality of the skin.

A note of caution

If you are already using Retin A cream, let your dermatologist know about it; or simply stay away from any extra procedures, as you probably won't need them anyway. The Retin A promotes new skin growth by stimulating the epidermis layer, so any more skin renewal treatment would be too much. Generally, if you use Retin A in conjunction with an exfoliating cream once a week plus a good moisturizer, and eat good food and drink plenty of water, your skin will look great. The other alternative is to stop using Retin A a few weeks before having a peel done. Think carefully and choose wisely before you decide to get some work done to your skin, especially if it is already in good condition. Be grateful for what blessings you have!

CHEMICAL PEELS

Light, or so-called easy, peels can be done by anyone and may provide satisfactory results for many people. They contain varying strengths of citric acid, which is sometimes all that is required. The medical-grade peels are more invasive; they have a recovery period of two to three weeks while the new skin regenerates. One should be prepared for some discomfort, as these peels are like a severe sunburn. Peels can produce good results for people with altered pigmentation or marked acne scarring.

Light peels can help to clear accumulated dead skin cells, acne, freckles, liver spots, and uneven skin texture. There are all sorts of peels available, but only the lighter peels should be undertaken at a spa or other similar establishments. Heavier peels should be performed by a cosmetic doctor. The end result is smooth skin—which may be slightly pink, but this can be rectified with a little foundation until full healing has occurred. This type of treatment needs to be repeated about once a month, with follow up sessions every two to three months.

Medium and heavier peels are stronger in effect and therefore take more time to heal. Expect some peeling of the skin, ranging from mild to severe. The heavier the peel is, the more peeling occurs on the skin. This would go from a sun-burned looking face for about a week, to a more burned look going from brown to pink over a two-week period, before the new skin is revealed. The latter treatment would only be done once a year at the most, and some recuperation time needs to be taken, as the peeling can be quite unsightly.

A very deep peel would only be done once in a lifetime. It is performed under anesthetic, and it is a really drastic measure undertaken for extremely damaged skins only. It takes several months before the final results can be seen. Serious research and deep thinking must be done before considering this kind of treatment.

Lasers are popular today and there are many kinds to choose from. Some lasers have similar effects to those described for chemical peels. The skin is basically being "polished" (a little bit like sandpaper on wood), which stimulates a newer version of itself to grow. The materials used range from salt crystals to powered diamonds. Lasers have grown in popularity against chemical peels as they seem to provoke far less adverse reactions. Laser treatments are also available in different strength categories.

Other lasers include pigment lasers; these are best suited for liver spots and should only be done once, assuming that subsequent good care is taken to avoid further sun exposure.

Vascular Lasers are used to remove birthmarks and rosacea (broken capillaries). The procedure can be repeated as required.

Microdermabrasion is similar to a light acid peel and can be used once a month. The skin may be a little raw after the treatment, but if a good *natural* moisturizer is used afterward, it will heal rapidly.

Dermabrasion is a heavier version of the above, leaving the skin quite raw for about two to four weeks. It could take several months for you to enjoy seeing the final results. This is done once every one to two years.

An alternative to all the above treatments

Light therapy can contribute to healing most skin conditions named above, although it works relatively slowly. This treatment does not cause the skin to peel off to renew itself, but many sessions are needed to start seeing some results. The side effects are practically nonexistent.

Important note: *Wear SPF every day.* This is essential, especially if you are using any kind of skin resurfacing methods. You will get all your liver spots back and more if you don't.

LIST OF QUESTIONS FOR ALL COSMETIC PROCEDURES

This list is designed to help you ask your cosmetic doctor all the information you need to know to make informed decisions.

- What qualifications does your chosen doctor have?
- Is there a personal consultation; is it free of charge or what is the cost?
- What amount of treatment is required to obtain full and final results?
- What is the *entire* cost of the procedure?
- What is the length of time of each treatment?
- Is there anything you can do to prepare your skin before treatments?
- What level of discomfort is to be expected, if any?
- What results can be expected according to your own skin quality and texture, based on their experience with previous clients?

- What are the side effects, if any?
- Do they provide effective support to remedy serious side effects?
- How much time is needed for side effects to subside?
- How long will it take for your skin to look its best again?
- How long can you expect the benefits of each treatment to last?

Notes: Find the most qualified and experienced practitioner possible. As mentioned previously, word of mouth and reputation are the best ways to find the professional you need. Once you find someone you are satisfied with, keep him/her! Reputable clinics do not charge for consultations.

If things are unclear and you are not satisfied with the level of information and care provided, find someone else. There are plenty of professional establishments that will not mind you being inquisitive; it is your face after all! Do not feel obliged to go ahead with any procedures, even if pre-booked, unless you are feeling *absolutely at peace* with your decision.

TOPICS EXPLORED IN SECTION 3

- Are skin peels necessary for you?
- A look at different peeling methods
- Indispensable list of questions to take to your cosmetic doctor/surgeon before committing to any procedures

NOTES

4. Cosmetic Surgery

A FEW WORDS OF CAUTION

At the risk of repeating myself, I will say once more that finding the best professional you can is *more than crucial*. Cosmetic surgery is to be taken as seriously as any other surgery. Some of the risks incurred are the very same as those of a medical operation; once you go under full anesthetic, many risks are present. An ethical and highly professional doctor will enquire about your full medical history, both physical and mental, before proceeding any further. Your reasons for wanting such an operation should be serious enough. You must consider all the risks involved with full knowledge and acute awareness before going ahead with any procedure. *The list of questions on page 268 must absolutely be used before booking any procedures.*

Add the following question to that list:

- What can I expect with this procedure as the body and/or the skin ages? ***Very important!***

Some people prefer to travel away for their cosmetic operations; different countries offer competitive prices, but this is really at your own risk. Give this some careful consideration, as you will probably have to travel again for checkup visits; or you may wish to know that you have the security of local support in case you suffer from side effects. Not having a local support system at your disposal may prove difficult and be a source of worry and stress, neither of which are conducive to healing. You may also need a second operation to touch up the work done the first time. So although traveling away for your cosmetic procedure may sound attractive (because of the prices offered), you should consider the convenience and safety factors involved with such a choice.

There are an astonishing number of physical alterations available today. I am not going to cover them all here; my aim is simply to share some information on a few of the most popular interventions, which I hope you will find useful if you are considering having anything done.

COSMETIC INTERVENTION ON YOUNG PEOPLE

Ladies

If you are a young woman, and are dealing with a doctor who will do any physical alterations you want (and on top of that, recommends that you do more than you requested, which happens, unfortunately), you are being completely misled. If you are in your twenties, your body is still changing and growing, and you will probably end up regretting your decision later. If you are planning on having cosmetic surgery done *before* your early twenties, *please reconsider*. The fact that today's society has you believing that plastic surgery done at such an early age is acceptable *is actual insanity,* and is usually promoted by unscrupulous, greedy individuals who make their fortune on your back. Your life's path will change, and choices made at an earlier stage of your life may become a burden. You might feel that you are sure of yourself and that you know exactly what you want, but I can tell you that there is only one thing that I am really sure about, which is that everything changes, especially our minds!

This generation has the most choices available to them in the way of physical alterations. You are being visually and mentally assaulted by the media on a daily basis with unrealistic images of what beauty is *meant* to look like, which is really tough on you. Your emotions are based on unrealistic mental projections, belonging to someone else. You have a tall order: letting your natural wisdom prevail at an early age, when all you want to do is experience as much as you can, which is the natural tendency of youth. I hope that you can find it in yourself to listen to your inner guidance and act with the strength you have, which is necessary to keep yourself free from obvious and completely unnecessary harm.

Consider this:

- Wait a few years—after having had your children for example; your breasts, tummy, and bottom may really need it by then!
- You may want children later on in your life, so breast implants are not a good choice early on, as your breast size increases up to three times during pregnancy. That means they will drop even more later on!
- You might not be able to breastfeed your baby with breast implants, and you may regret that once you have your little gem in your arms looking at you with all the love in the world.
- You might lose partial or total sensation of the whole breast and/or nipples, for life … a great shame!

GENITAL COSMETIC SURGERY

Gentlemen

For those of you young men (and all others) who are considering having genital cosmetic surgery hoping for a larger penis, consider this: it is better to have one that functions well and that you know how to use, rather than a floppy friend for life! I would like to add that there is absolutely no sarcasm intended here, just some care and real concern. There are a few places in life where size is simply not worth considering, and this is definitely one of them. The risks are too great. Besides, being a good lover and pleasing your partner have absolutely nothing to do with size. Please check out pages 195-210 where we explore sexual ecstasy, and have a look at books in the recommended list of reading (3, 10, 11, and 12).

Ladies

Do some serious thinking before you even consider having anything done to enhance your sexual pleasure through the use of plastic surgery. At least do yourself a favor and research other ways to improve and increase your orgasms *first.* You owe it to yourself. Look into Taoist and Tantric practices to work on developing a more intimate connection with yourself and your partner. Do you know that you have access to *unlimited pleasure* and that you can orgasm many times consecutively if you want to? Genital cosmetic surgery has only been performed recently and we simply do not have enough data to make a decent evaluation of all the possible side effects. What we know is that there may be a loss of sensation in the vulva or clitoris, temporary or permanent. Think of a life without orgasms ... it is considerably worse than chocolate cake without the chocolate!

Note: The practice of clitoral mutilation is still performed in certain countries today. This is a sad and disempowering reality of which many women are victims. Why take a risk to lose your God-given access to ecstasy? See pages 195-210 to gain information regarding the expansion of your own sexuality, and read a book or two from the recommended list of reading: (2, 3, and 11). Also check out the PC exercises on pages 212-122.

ON A MORE GENERAL NOTE

Plastic surgery *only* improves the way you look—not how you feel

Cosmetic surgery, in general, is exclusively for your own benefit; it should be discreet enough so others do not notice it. It is important to realize that plastic surgery will not fix any problems in your relationships, whether they are ones you are having with yourself or with someone else.

Do not expect to get *automatic self-confidence*; this is only gained with work done by yourself, on yourself. However, if you are fully aware of all the facts regarding a particular procedure and still want to go ahead, I invite you to meditate on your decision and to *wait* until you feel completely sure before having anything done. This could take anything from a few days to several months, or even a year or more; there should be no rush when considering having permanent alterations done to your face or body. If something does not feel right, or if you are hesitant about your decision, consider postponing the surgery until you feel clearer about your choices. The hesitation you feel could be your inner guidance warning you that something will not work out, or that you will experience side effects you might not be able to cope with. I hope that by you are now able to listen to your own intuition and to trust what you feel.

Remember that doubt means no.

However, cosmetic surgery can be appropriate and, in some cases, change someone's life in an entirely positive way. *It is both daunting and fascinating to know that we can "order" our body parts to look different.* When used in moderation and with discretion, it can have a beneficial effect. In some extreme cases, plastic surgery can enhance a person's life, providing that the physical transformation is accompanied by some self-development, ensuring that self-confidence is real and permanent.

Breast implants

This is probably the most practiced cosmetic procedure today. Here are some facts to bear in mind:

- There may be a loss of sensation in the breast and/or nipples, temporary or permanent.
- Most of us are asymmetrical; the implants are not. You may notice the difference once the implants are in, but it is usually only noticeable by yourself. If the asymmetry is very pronounced, you can request a different size implant in one of your breasts.

- Consider what kind of sport you do and make sure that your choice will not impede your ability to carry on as usual.
- Bear in mind that lying comfortably on your front is probably not going to be an option any more, especially on a hard surface.

A word of caution

An important fact to consider is that, as the skin ages, the implant will pull the skin of the breast down because it is heavier; and you eventually get a "ball-in-sock" effect. Give this some consideration before choosing the size and, therefore, the weight of your implants. A good doctor will use something that is in natural proportion with your body. The obvious and best candidates for this operation (besides medical reasons such as mastectomy following breast cancer) are mothers who have finished breastfeeding all their children and want to regain their original shape, or after extreme weight loss.

Liposuction is best done while the elasticity of the skin is at its maximum, which would be before the age of thirty-five. If this is done later, the skin that is covering the area where the cellulite used to be will not fully "bounce back" and will therefore sag as a result. This often looks worse than the initial problem. If the sagging is severe, more surgery can be performed to remove excess skin; but if you don't fancy looking like patchwork, this option is not worth considering. *Cellulite never killed anyone; but too much surgery can certainly do a lot of damage.* Also note that liposuction is best used to remove deposits that cannot be gotten rid of with weight loss. Many slim people have cellulite and they all seem to be female. You, gentlemen, have problems of your own apparently, but not this one!

Cellulite: No bother!

After doing some extensive research on the subject, I am very glad to announce that *most men don't mind cellulite*! Yes, that is what a majority of men say. This means that the only people who have a problem with it are women; and when you think of it, it's not really that bad—there are worst fates in life! If your man doesn't mind it, you can either accept it or cover it up cleverly when you choose an outfit It only leaves you with a small challenge at the beach when you are on holidays. Don't worry: you probably won't know anyone this far away from home!

Tip: The pineapple tip in the Restylane section on page 261 is very useful for post-liposuction, as there usually is a *huge amount* of bruising at the site of the operation. Eat a small amount of pineapple two to three times a day to dramatically decrease the bruising.

Facial cosmetic alterations are some of the most delicate surgeries you can have done, as your face is the most exposed part of your body. Thankfully, the time of ridiculously out-of-proportion features has *almost* passed, as more and more surgeons favor decisions that are complementary to the client's features and personality. There are unfortunately some exceptions to this, owing to greedy and unethical practitioners; so, once again, it is up to you to be vigilant if you want to get some surgical cosmetic work done.

Tips:

- If any of the bones were worked on during one of many possible cosmetic operations, comfrey cream applied topically helps the bone tissue to re-knit promptly. It can be used several times a day, as soon as it can be applied directly over the bone that received the operation.
- Drinking comfrey tea is equally useful, and in fact a great deal more practical, especially if you are wearing a plaster cast. It yields wonderful results any time that the bones have been fractured, whether you have had cosmetic work

done or have a broken limb. It contributes to the bone re-knitting itself and to the healing of soft tissue; it is so powerful that you must make sure the bone is set properly (in the case of a broken limb) before you drink this tea.

- Eating calcium-rich foods will also speed up and promote the healing process. Choose from: porridge, dates, cheese, milk, tofu, salmon, sardines, eggs, spinach, beans, almonds, etc.

Facelifts are a last resort, as there are plenty of ways to keep yourself looking your best without such a serious surgical intervention. We have explored many natural methods to keep yourself looking and feeling your best in the first four chapters. New alternatives to facelifts are constantly being updated; thread-lifts are the least invasive equivalent available today.

The best time to have a facelift, if you have already made up your mind to do so, is in your late forties or early fifties. The golden rule is to *wait as long as possible* before getting this done; any ethical cosmetic doctor will tell you that *no facelift should be done before the age of forty*. Facelifts should only be done twice in a person's lifetime, at the very most—that is, if you want natural-looking results; once only would be better still. Remember that the skin is not elastic forever, and the static look one gets from having had too much surgery is not particularly attractive.

Remember that you are already beautiful!

5. Aging Gracefully

There is a difference between wanting to look your best for as long as possible and not accepting aging at all. Aging happens to us whether we like it or not, and giving it negative attention only makes it a bigger hurdle to get over.

The beauty that emanates from you comes from within.

Do you ever catch yourself so fascinated when connecting with someone that you barely notice what they wear, what hair-do they have, or how old they might be ... and yet you find that person quite beautiful?

Your body is the house of your soul

True contentment arises when your body and your soul are aware of one another and cohabitate with love, peace, and respect.

I wish you well on your journey toward yourself.
May you feel present and at peace,
may you feel beautiful and powerful,
for you are the Creator's manifested choice!
I wish you laugher, love, joy,
and all other kinds of prosperity
that are Divinely intended for you.
Take care of yourself with as much attention and passion
as you would give your lover.
There is only one of you,
you matter to us all.
Your contribution is valued and appreciated,
We are all ONE.

With Love and Peace beyond all understanding,

Mahayana

TOPICS EXPLORED IN SECTION 4

- A word of caution regarding cosmetic surgery
- Cosmetic intervention on young people
- A look at popular cosmetic surgeries
- Tips for recovery and side effects of cosmetic surgery
- Aging gracefully

NOTES

APPENDIX

Space for Your Dreams and Goals

1. A list of the things I want to change

2. My monthly goals and achievements

3. My yearly goals and achievements

Exercises and Rituals

Recipes

BIBLIOGRAPHY

(1.) Airola, Paavo. Worldwide Secrets for Staying Young. Scottsdale, Arizona: Health Plus Publishers, 1982.

(2.) Anand, Margot. The Art of Every Day Ecstasy. New York: Random House, 1998.

(3.) ———. The Art of Sexual Ecstasy. New York: Penguin Putnam, Inc., 1989.

(4.) Armstrong, John W. The Water of Life. United Kingdom: Vermilion Publishing, 2005.

(5.) Batmanghelidj, F. Water for Health, for Healing, for Life. New York: Warner Books, Inc., 1992.

(6.) Batt, Eva. Vegan Cooking. Wellingborough, England: Thorsons Publishers, 1985.

(7.) Breuss, Rudolph. The Breuss Cancer Cure. Burnaby, British Columbia: Books Alive, 1998.

(8.) Burroughs, Stanley. The Master Cleanser. Burroughs Books, 1976.

(9.) Canfield, Jack. The Success Principles. Harper Paperbacks, 2006.

(10.) Chang, Stephen T. The Complete System of Self-Healing: Internal Exercises. London: Tao Publishing, 1984.

(11.) ———. The Tao of Sexology, The Book of Infinite Wisdom. London: Tao Publishing, 1986.

(12.) Chia, Mantak. Cultivating Male Sexual Energy. Harper Collins Inc., 1996.

(13.) Davis, Patricia. Aromatherapy, an A-Z. Essex, United Kingdom: C. W. Daniel Co., Ltd., 1988.

(14.) ———. Subtle Aromatherapy. Essex, United Kingdom: C. W. Daniel Co., Ltd., 1991.

(15.) Gelb, Michael. Body Learning. New York: Henry Holt and Company, LLC, 1981.

(16.) Hall, Judy. The Crystal Bible. London: Octopus Publishing Group, 2009.

(17.) Hendrix, Harville. Getting the Love You Want. New York: Henry Holt and Company, LLC., 1998.

(18.) Kenton, Leslie. Passage to Power. USA: Hay House, Inc., 1998.
(19.) Kroom, Coen van der. The Golden Fountain. Mesa, Arizona: Amethyst Books, 1996.
(20.) Lawless, Julia. The Encyclopedia of Essential Oils. London: Element Books, 1995.
(21.) Lipton, Bruce H. The Biology of Belief. United Kingdom: Hay House Inc., 2008.
(22.) McIntyre, Anne. Healing Drinks. London: Gaia Book Ltd., 2000.
(23.) McTaggart, Lynne. The Intention Experiment. London: Harper Element, 2007.
(24.) Mello, Anthony de. A Call to Love. India: Sahitatya Prakash, 1991.
(25.) Pert, Candace. Molecules of Emotion. New York: Scribner, 1997.
(26.) Robbins, Anthony. Unlimited Power. New York: Free Press, 2003.
(27.) Roeder, Dorothy. Crystals Co-Creators. Sedona, Arizona: Light Technology Publishing, 1994.
(28.) Shaw, Miranda. Passionate Enlightenment. Princeton, New Jersey: Princeton University Press, 1994.
(29.) Smith, Robin L. Lies at the Altar. New York: Hyperion, 2006.
(30.) Snodgrass, Edmund and Lucie. Green Roof Plants: A Resource and Planting Guide. Portland, Oregon: Timber Press, Inc., 2006.
(31.) Tolle, Eckhart. A New Earth. London: Penguin Group, 2005.
(32.) ———. The Power of Now. Novato, California: New World Library, 1999.
(33.) Wheater, Caroline. Juicing for Health/The Juicing Detox Diet. Wellingborough, England: Thorsons Publishers, 1993.

INDEX

A

B

F

G

H

I

J

K

L

M

U

V

W

Y

Lightning Source UK Ltd.
Milton Keynes UK
174075UK00001B/56/P

9 781609 768997